28-DAY CHALLENGE

WALL PILATES

for SENIORS

2024

200+ ILLUSTRATIONS

100+ VIDEOS

🎁 3 BONUS

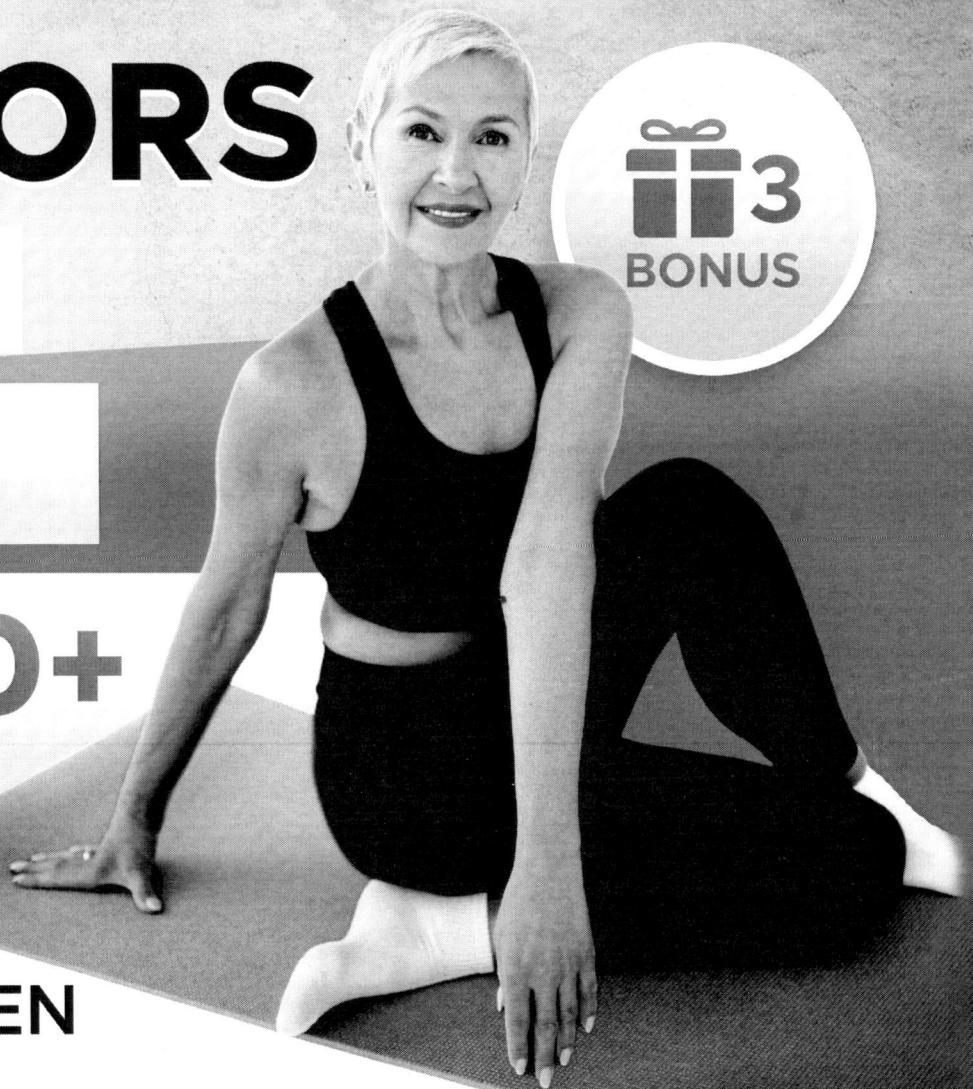

GRACE NOREN

Summary Index

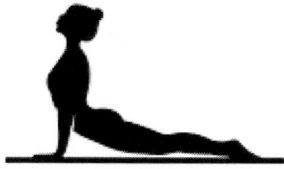

Chapter 1:
Foreword

"Every moment of our life can be the beginning of great things."

Joseph Pilates

1.1 – Introduction to Wall Pilates

Introducing Wall Pilates, a revolutionary technique that is changing the way we think about health and vitality as we age. A creative twist on the classic Pilates method, wall Pilates was created to enable seniors to reap the many health advantages of this training regimen regardless of their degree of mobility or physical fitness. In addition to guaranteeing safety and stability, this technique allows seniors to participate in a fulfilling training program by using a wall for support while performing a variety of activities.

Even though the phrase "Wall Pilates" is relatively new, it is based on ideas that Joseph Pilates first presented in the early 1900s. With an emphasis on control, accuracy, and fluid movements, Joseph Pilates developed Pilates as a type of exercise to improve the body and mind. **Pilates exercises have evolved to include wall support as a modern adaptation to make the practice more accessible to a larger range of people, including the elderly and those with limited mobility.** Modern Pilates teachers and physical therapists who saw the need for a more flexible and secure exercise option for senior citizens are attributed with the development and spread of Wall Pilates as a distinct practice. It's a great option for anyone who might find standard Pilates mats or equipment scary or difficult because it allows practitioners to focus on movement correctness, maintain balance more readily, and lower their risk of injury.

Traditional Pilates is not the same as Wall Pilates in numerous important aspects. Numerous exercises are performed on a mat or with specific apparatus in traditional Pilates. A certain amount of core strength, flexibility, and balance are required for these workouts. By using the wall as a tool for support, alignment, and resistance, Wall Pilates, on the other hand, streamlines the methodology. The same fundamental Pilates principles—breath control, centering, attention, and precision—may be emphasized with this adaptation, which also makes accommodations for potential age-related physical limits or difficulties.

Through the use of tactile input from the wall, practitioners are assisted in maintaining appropriate alignment and posture during each exercise. In addition, it provides resistance akin to that of Pilates apparatus, facilitating muscular building via application of force against the wall. **Because of its versatility,**

Wall Pilates is particularly helpful for senior citizens, offering a safer setting to increase flexibility, strengthen the core, and improve general fitness without running the danger of strain or injury.

Through deliberate breathing and deliberate movement execution, Wall Pilates not only enhances physical health but also mental and emotional wellness. It promotes calm and stress relief by promoting a meditative state. This all-encompassing approach to wellness emphasizes the practice's attraction and makes it an appealing option for anyone looking to add strength, balance, and peace to their latter years. Are you prepared to start a new chapter in your health with Wall Pilates? Age is nothing more than a number when it comes to pursuing and preserving health and energy, as demonstrated by this practice. Allow Wall Pilates to lead you to a more lively, harmonious, and contented life.

1.2 – Staying Active: A Key to Vitality

How come maintaining an active lifestyle becomes both a challenge and a must as we approach our elderly years? Not only should physical health be sought after, but a deeply meaningful life full of energy, meaning, and happiness is the key to the solution. Frequent exercise, like the increasingly well-liked Wall Pilates method, is a ray of hope for senior citizens, offering an interesting and life-changing route to improved wellbeing.

For seniors who want to preserve their independence, improve their health, and fully enjoy life, wall Pilates in particular has become essential. As a nourishing journey for the body, mind, and spirit, this practice goes beyond the typical confines of exercise. Each participant will be able to go out on a journey of renewal and exploration in the comfort and safety of their surroundings thanks to this comprehensive approach to wellbeing.

What then makes Wall Pilates the best option for older adults? The response is complex. To begin with, it respects and honors the body's current state while gently promoting growth in balance, strength, and flexibility—all important aspects of fall prevention and an active lifestyle. Every movement and stretch is infused with confidence since the wall is a steady companion, providing support and stability that greatly reduces the chance of damage.

Wall Pilates has many advantages beyond its physical aspects, though. Additionally, mental health might find refuge in this exercise. It reduces stress and soothes tension while igniting a sense of calm and emotional balance via focused breathing and purposeful movement. A calm perspective on life's ups and downs is bestowed upon practitioners by this gift of mental clarity, which elevates the quality of existence.

Because Wall Pilates can be customized to meet individual needs, no two sessions are ever the same thanks to its versatility. **Wall Pilates facilitates inclusivity and adaptability by providing a range of alternatives, from a standing stretch that helps with posture correction to a leg workout that bolsters the lower body while supported by the wall.**

However, Wall Pilates is more than simply a set of exercises; it's an invitation to investigate the mutually beneficial link between the body and mind, to accept and be grateful for every moment of the present, and to celebrate every accomplishment, no matter how small. It advocates for living an active lifestyle in our latter years, which adds life to our days rather than just more days.

A daily practice that incorporates Wall Pilates is a statement of one's dedication to live life to the fullest, pushing the envelope of what's possible, and dispelling myths about aging. This demonstrates the unwavering determination of those who choose to define themselves not by the years they have lived but rather by the breadth and depth of their experiences.

1.3 – How This Book Can Help You

With a guide designed for transformation as much as for exercise, discover the vast world of Wall Pilates. Regardless of your experience level or current fitness level, this book is a carefully crafted trip that is suited to meet you where you are. It is not a one-size-fits-all. This guide will be your constant companion on your journey to improved health and vitality, regardless of whether you're just starting out or looking to intensify your current fitness routine.

Tailored to Individual Needs: Understanding that everyone has a different starting place when it comes to fitness, this guide provides a range of exercises suitable for beginners as well as those looking to improve on an already established practice. It shows that the understanding that customization is essential to accessibility in physical exercise is present.

Caters to a Variety of Goals: Understanding that there are many different reasons people practice Wall Pilates—from wanting to gain more strength and flexibility to wanting assistance with weight loss—the book has parts specifically designed to address these varied objectives. This guarantees that you will receive help and direction according to your needs, regardless of your goal.

Holistic Approach to Wellness: This book promotes a holistic approach to wellbeing that goes beyond physical fitness and includes activities that enhance mental and emotional well-being in addition to physical fitness. Recognizing the connection between the mind, body, and spirit, this all-encompassing approach provides a route to wellbeing that honors the individual as a whole.

Supportive of All Ages: Even though the book is primarily written with seniors in mind, all age groups can benefit from its universally helpful principles and practices. This book's dedication to creating a community where anybody interested in Wall Pilates may find value and support is highlighted by its diversity.

This book serves as a call to action, motivating you to use Wall Pilates as a tool to improve your physical state regardless of your starting point.

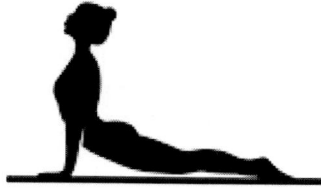

CHAPTER 2:
GETTING STARTED

"In 10 sessions, you'll feel the difference, in 20 sessions you'll see the difference, and in 30 sessions you'll have a whole new body."

Joseph Pilates

It takes careful planning ahead and a deep comprehension of the fundamentals of Wall Pilates to begin. The next parts will go into more detail about how to set up your practice area, get the tools you need, put safety precautions in place, and sharpen your focus.

2.1 – Setting Up Your Practice Space

Creating a dedicated and conducive space for your Wall Pilates practice is essential in fostering an environment that supports your journey to wellness. Here's how to craft a special corner in your home into a haven for your Pilates sessions:

Selecting Your Space:

- **Quiet Area:** Find a peaceful section of your home where distractions are few. A tranquil environment encourages concentration and inner peace during your practice.

- **Space Requirements:** Ensure the chosen area has enough wall space for support and is free from obstructions. You'll need sufficient room to extend your arms, legs, and to perform movements against the wall comfortably.

Lighting:

- **Natural Light:** Ideally, position your practice space near a window. Natural sunlight not only elevates your mood but also keeps you attuned to the day's natural flow.

- **Artificial Lighting:** In darker spaces, choose soft, ambient artificial lighting. Warm, adjustable lighting can help create a calming atmosphere, enhancing your Pilates experience.

Flooring:

- **Stable Surface:** A solid, level floor is vital for safety and effectiveness. Hardwood floors are ideal, providing the firmness needed for exercises.

- **Non-slip Solutions:** If practicing on slick surfaces, a high-quality, non-slip mat placed against the wall can secure your stance and protect against sliding.

Personal Touches:

- **Inspirational Items:** Personalize your space with items that inspire serenity and motivation, such as vibrant indoor plants, motivational quotes, or art that resonates with your spirit.

- **Comfort Additions:** Enhance your space with a few comforts like a plush mat for standing exercises or a soft towel for support during various poses.

Organizational Tips:

- **Storage Solutions:** Keep essential Pilates accessories, like resistance bands or small weights, within reach. A neatly organized shelf or storage bin can prevent clutter and keep your practice area orderly.

- **Space Clearance:** Maintain a minimalist setup by decluttering regularly. A clean and open space can significantly reduce stress, promoting a more focused and effective practice.

Atmospheric Enhancements:

- **Aromatherapy:** Introduce calming aromas with essential oil diffusers or scented candles. Scents like lavender or peppermint can relax the mind and enhance concentration.

- **Soundscapes:** Soft background music or nature sounds can help in creating a more immersive and relaxing practice environment, allowing you to delve deeper into your Wall Pilates routine.

By using these well considered tips to set up your Wall Pilates practice area, you're creating a holistic haven that supports your body and mind in addition to a physical area for training. Your journey toward health and vitality is enhanced by this committed setting, which encourages a deeper involvement with your practice.

2.2 – Essential Equipment

- **A Sturdy Wall:** Central to Wall Pilates, a sturdy, clear wall space is indispensable. It serves as your primary support for a variety of exercises, enabling you to perform movements with precision and safety. Choose a wall that is free from obstructions and decorations, ensuring enough space for exercises that involve full body extensions, leaning, and pushing movements.

- **Non-slip Mat:** A high-quality, non-slip mat is crucial for providing stability and cushioning during your practice. This mat will lie on the floor to prevent slipping and to protect your body during floor exercises. It also serves as a marker of your personal practice space, helping to define the area where you'll perform your Wall Pilates routines.

- **Comfortable Attire:** The right clothing can make a significant difference in your Pilates practice. Opt for attire that is breathable, allowing for optimal airflow to keep you cool. It should also offer stretchability to accommodate the wide range of movements in Wall Pilates, from stretches to more dynamic exercises. Your clothing should be snug enough to allow your instructor or yourself to observe your movements and ensure proper form, but not so tight as to restrict any movement.

2.3 – Safety Tips and Modifications

Starting a Wall Pilates practice entails not just picking up new moves but also making sure you perform them correctly and safely. Here are some vital pointers to remember, beginning with the important warm-up and adding a fresh suggestion for keeping a secure and effective practicing space.

1. **Warm-Up:**

   - **Gradual Preparation:** Begin your session with a series of gentle stretches and movements that prepare your body for the workout ahead. Warming up increases your heart rate and blood flow to muscles, reducing the risk of injury.

   - **Specific Exercises:** Focus on warm-up exercises that activate the core, as well as the muscles you'll be using during your session. Wall slides, arm circles, and gentle squats against the wall can effectively prepare your body for more intensive Pilates work.

2. **Listening to Your Body:**

   - **Self-awareness:** Monitor how your body responds to each exercise. If you feel any discomfort or pain, modify the movement or stop altogether.

   - **Respecting Limits:** Acknowledge your body's capabilities, which can vary daily, and adjust your practice accordingly to prevent strain.

3. **Gradual Progression:**

   - **Start with the Basics:** Initiate your practice with foundational poses, focusing on proper form and breathing.

   - **Incremental Challenges:** Gradually incorporate more advanced poses to build strength and flexibility without risking injury.

4. **Utilizing Props:**

   - **Adaptability:** Employ props such as cushions or resistance bands to make exercises more accessible and comfortable.

   - **Creative Support:** In absence of traditional props, household items can be effective substitutes, like towels for straps.

5. **Maintaining Focus:**

   - **Concentration on Movement and Breath:** Engage deeply with your body's movements and your breathing to enhance focus and prevent mishaps.

   - **Mindful Transitions:** Transition carefully between exercises to avoid injuries, which are more likely during these moments.

6. **Hydration:**

   - **Regular Intake:** Stay hydrated before, during, and after your practice. Keep water close at hand during your session.

   - **Listen to Thirst Cues:** Heed your body's signals for water, especially under warm conditions or during longer workouts.

7. **Space Safety:**

   - **Clear Area:** Ensure your practice space is free of obstacles that could cause trips or falls.

   - **Secure Environment:** Confirm that your practice surface is stable and secure, using mats or rugs to prevent slips.

8. **Personal Comfort:**

   - **Appropriate Attire:** Choose clothes that allow unrestricted movement and won't distract or discomfort you.

   - **Room Temperature:** Keep the practice area at a comfortable temperature to help maintain focus and proper hydration levels.

9. **Enhancing Body Alignment:**

   - **Postural Awareness:** Throughout your practice, remain cognizant of your body's alignment. Proper alignment is key to executing Wall Pilates exercises effectively and safely.

   - **Alignment Checks:** Regularly pause to assess and adjust your posture, ensuring that your spine is aligned, your core is engaged, and your movements are controlled and precise.

2.4 – How to Enhancing Your Focus in 8 Steps

Any Pilates practice, including Wall Pilates, must be based on focus. It connects the dots between movement and consciousness, transforming each practice into a kind of meditation. Exercises that require a high level of focus increase the mind-body connection and help people move more precisely, balance better, and have a better understanding of their own bodies.

Hereafter 8 Strategies for Enhancing Focus.

1. **Create a Distraction-Free Environment:** Before beginning your practice, ensure your space is conducive to concentration. A tidy, quiet area free of distractions allows you to fully immerse yourself in the session. Consider turning off electronic devices or using them solely for playing soft, instrumental music that fosters concentration.

2. **Set Clear Intentions:** Starting your practice with a clear intention can significantly improve focus. Whether it's improving posture, enhancing flexibility, or simply dedicating time to self-care, having a specific goal in mind directs your attention and energy towards achieving it.

3. **Employ Mindful Breathing**: Breathing techniques are at the heart of Pilates. Focusing on your breath helps anchor your attention in the present moment, facilitating a deeper connection with your body. Practice deep, controlled breathing to initiate movement, using the rhythm of your breath to maintain focus throughout your session.

4. **Visualize the Movements:** Before executing each exercise, take a moment to visualize the movement in your mind. This mental rehearsal not only prepares the body for the physical activity but also sharpens focus, making each movement more intentional and effective.

5. **Limit the Length of Sessions:** Longer sessions can lead to mental fatigue, reducing the quality of your practice. Keep your Wall Pilates sessions concise, especially in the beginning. A focused 20-minute session is more beneficial than an hour of distracted exercise.

6. **Incorporate Mindfulness Practices:** Integrate mindfulness techniques into your routine. Between exercises, take brief moments to connect with your senses, observing any sensations, emotions, or thoughts without judgment. This practice enhances overall focus and brings a sense of calmness to your workout.

7. **Regularly Change Your Routine:** Varying your exercise routine prevents mental stagnation and keeps the practice engaging. Introducing new exercises or variations challenges the body and mind, requiring renewed focus and learning.

8. **Reflect Post-Session:** After completing your session, spend a few minutes reflecting on the practice. Acknowledge the moments of strong focus and consider the areas where your mind wandered. This reflection is crucial for understanding your patterns of attention and devising strategies for improvement.

To get the most out of Wall Pilates and maximize its benefits, one must pay close attention at all times. Recall that wall Pilates is a mindfulness practice that calls for perseverance, commitment, and, most importantly, concentrated attention. It's not just a physical workout.

2.5 – 8 Common Mistakes to Avoid

It is important to be aware of typical mistakes when doing wall Pilates, especially if you are an older practitioner, as these can impede your progress or cause injury. You can guarantee a safer, more productive workout by being aware of these errors:

1. **Ignoring Proper Alignment:** Wall Pilates relies heavily on your body's alignment against the wall. Misalignment, such as slouching or tilting your pelvis, can strain your muscles and joints. Always start by checking your alignment – your head, shoulders, hips, and heels should be in a straight line against the wall.

2. **Overextending the Neck:** During exercises, there's a tendency to strain the neck, especially while trying to maintain a gaze on the mirror or checking your posture. This overextension can lead to neck pain. Focus on keeping your neck in a neutral position, aligned with your spine.

3. **Skipping Warm-Ups:** No matter your age, warming up is non-negotiable. As a senior, your muscles and joints require more time to become supple and ready for exercise. A gentle warm-up, such as walking in place or shoulder rolls, prepares your body and reduces the risk of injury.

4. **Pushing Too Hard:** It's easy to get carried away and push your body beyond its limits, especially when you start feeling more confident. However, pushing too hard can lead to muscle strains or more severe injuries. Listen to your body and recognize the difference between a challenging workout and overexertion.

5. **Neglecting Breath Control:** Pilates emphasizes the importance of breath control – inhaling and exhaling with movements. Incorrect breathing can increase blood pressure and reduce the effectiveness of your exercises. Practice inhaling deeply through your nose and exhaling slowly through your mouth.

6. **Forgetting to Hydrate:** Staying hydrated is essential, particularly for seniors. Dehydration can lead to dizziness and fatigue, making it harder to maintain focus and balance during your session. Keep a water bottle nearby and take small sips throughout your workout.

7. **Using Incorrect Footwear or Going Barefoot:** Proper footwear provides support and helps maintain balance. While some prefer the tactile feedback of going barefoot, supportive shoes can prevent slips and falls. Choose what works best for you, but ensure safety and comfort.

8. **Skipping Post-Workout Stretching:** After your wall Pilates session, stretching is vital. It helps to cool down your body, improve flexibility, and decrease muscle stiffness. Incorporate a few gentle stretches focusing on major muscle groups you've worked on.

IMPORTANT: HOW TO SEE THE VIDEOS

Next to the name of each exercise, you find a **QR code**.

Simply **SCAN** it with your smartphone and **CLICK ON THE LINK** displayed on your screen to watch the video where the instructor Jayni shows you exactly **HOW TO PERFORM** the exercise.

ABOUT THE INSTRUCTOR

Jayni is a friend of mine, an expert and passionate Yoga and Pilates instructor, whom I thank for her kindness and availability, and I admire for the great professionalism and passion with which she performs this wonderful job every day.

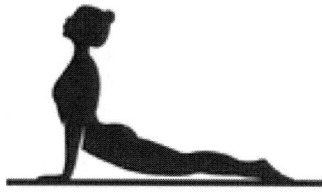

CHAPTER 3:
101 WALL PILATES EXERCISES

"Pilates is complete coordination of body, mind, and spirit."

Joseph Pilates

Are you prepared to set out on a path that goes beyond conventional fitness and provides a holistic approach to wellness? Allow this book to be your partner, your inspiration, and your guide as you work toward living a vibrant, resilient, and joyful life. Take the first steps toward transforming your life through movement by beginning your Wall Pilates journey right now.

3.1 – For Beginners

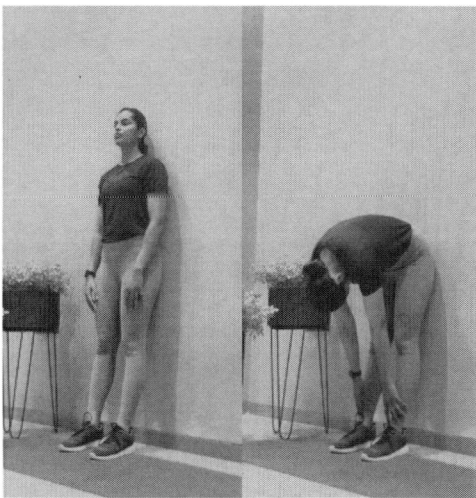

1.1 Wall Roll Down

Scan for Video!

- 🎯 **Objective:** Enhance spinal flexibility and release tension in the back.

- ◎ **Focus:** Back, shoulders.

- ⚓ **Position:** Stand with your back against the wall, feet shoulder-width apart.

- 💪 **Exercise:** Slowly roll down the wall by tucking the chin towards the chest and peeling the spine off the wall, one vertebra at a time. Go as low as comfortable.

- 🧍 **Breathing:** Inhale to start, exhale as you roll down.

⏱ **Time or Repetition:**

- Beginner: Roll down for 5 seconds, then back up.

- Intermediate: Roll down for 10 seconds, hold briefly, then back up.

- Advanced: Roll down for 15 seconds, hold briefly, then back up.

🧘 **Cool Down:** Gradually return to standing straight against the wall.

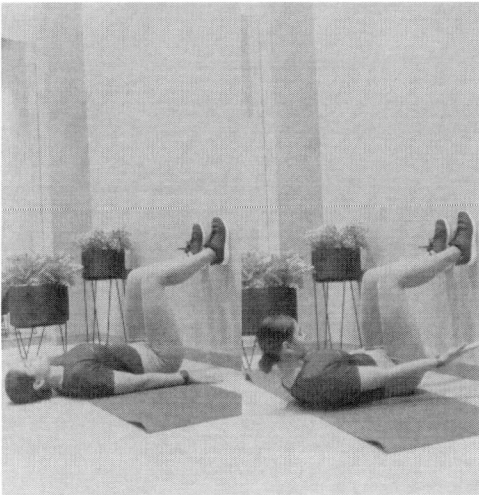

2. Wall Supported Hundred

Scan for Video!

🎯 **Objective:** Strengthen the core and improve respiratory system.

◎ **Focus:** Abdominals, breath control.

⚓ **Position:** Lie on your back with legs raised and bent at 90 degrees, arms extended along your sides, palms against the wall.

🏃 **Exercise:** Pump your arms up and down in small movements, breathing in for five pumps and out for five pumps.

🧘 **Breathing:** Inhale for five arm pumps, exhale for five arm pumps.

⏱ **Time or Repetition:**

- Beginner: 30 seconds.
- Intermediate: 45 seconds.
- Advanced: 60 seconds.

🧘 **Cool Down:** Slowly lower your legs and rest.

3. Wall Supported Bicycle

Scan for Video!

🎯 **Objective:** Enhance core strength and improve leg mobility.

◎ **Focus:** Core, legs.

⚓ **Position:** Lie on your back close to the wall, hands behind your head, legs raised to mimic a seated position.

🏃 **Exercise:** Alternate extending each leg as if pedaling a bicycle.

🧘 **Breathing:** Inhale as one leg extends, exhale as it returns.

⏱ **Time or Repetition:**

- Beginner: 30 seconds.
- Intermediate: 45 seconds.
- Advanced: 60 seconds.

🧘 **Cool Down:** Gently hug knees to chest and rock side to side.

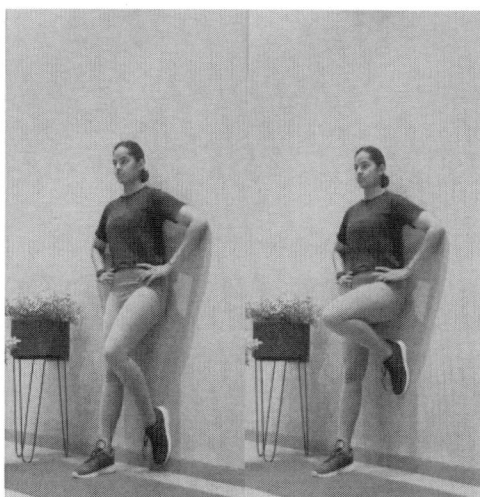

4. Wall Single Leg Slide

Scan for Video!

🎯 **Objective:** Improve lower body flexibility and strengthen the leg muscles.

◎ **Focus:** Legs, glutes.

⚓ **Position:** Stand with your back to the wall, feet hip-width apart. Place one foot slightly forward.

💪 **Exercise:** Slide the forward foot up the wall, then gently lower.

🧍 **Breathing:** Inhale as you slide up, exhale as you lower.

⏱ **Time or Repetition:**

- Beginner: 5 repetitions each leg.
- Intermediate: 8 repetitions each leg.
- Advanced: 10 repetitions each leg.

🧘 **Cool Down:** Stand tall, taking deep breaths.

5. Wall Standing Leg Circles

Scan for Video!

🎯 **Objective:** Increase hip mobility and improve balance.

◎ **Focus:** Hips, balance.

⚓ **Position:** Stand side-on to the wall, lightly touching it for balance. Extend the outside leg forward.

💪 **Exercise:** Circle the extended leg in small, controlled movements.

🧍 **Breathing:** Inhale to start, exhale during the circle.

⏱ **Time or Repetition:**

- Beginner: 5 circles each direction, each leg.
- Intermediate: 8 circles each direction, each leg.
- Advanced: 10 circles each direction, each leg.

🧘 **Cool Down:** Return to standing, switch sides.

14

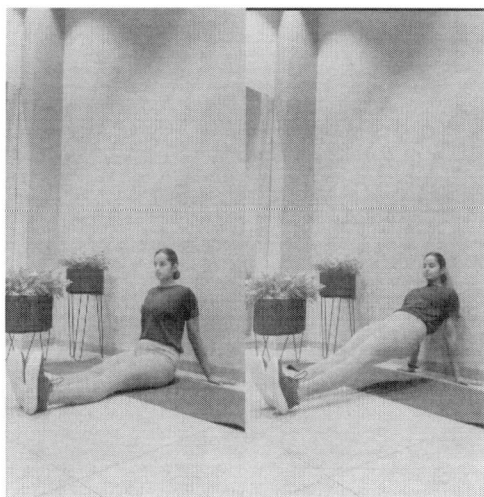

6. Wall Reverse Plank

Scan for Video!

◎ **Objective:** Strengthen the core, shoulders, and posterior chain.

◉ **Focus:** Core, shoulders, back.

⚓ **Position:** Sit facing away from the wall, legs extended, palms on the floor behind you, fingers pointing towards the wall.

🧘 **Exercise:** Lift your hips towards the ceiling, pressing your hands and heels into the floor.

🧍 **Breathing:** Inhale as you lift, exhale to hold.

⏱ **Time or Repetition:**

- Beginner: Hold for 10 seconds.

- Intermediate: Hold for 15 seconds.

- Advanced: Hold for 20 seconds.

🧘 **Cool Down:** Slowly lower your hips back to the floor.

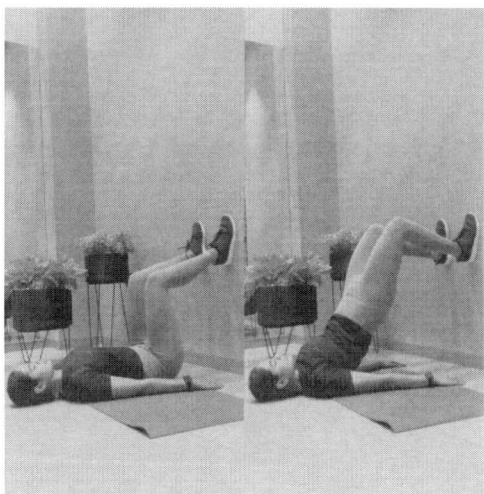

7. Wall Supported Bridge

Scan for Video!

◎ **Objective:** Enhance lower back strength and flexibility.

◉ **Focus:** Glutes, hamstrings, lower back.

⚓ **Position:** Lie on your back with feet flat against the wall, knees bent.

🧘 **Exercise:** Lift your hips towards the ceiling, forming a bridge.

🧍 **Breathing:** Inhale as you lift, exhale as you lower.

⏱ **Time or Repetition:**

- Beginner: Hold for 10 seconds.

- Intermediate: Hold for 15 seconds.

- Advanced: Hold for 20 seconds.

🧘 **Cool Down:** Gently roll the spine back to the floor.

15

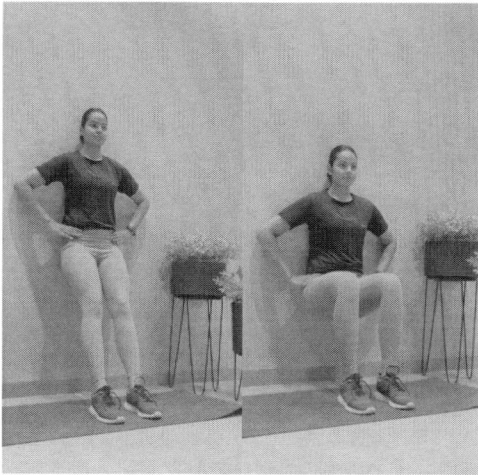

8. Deep Wall Sit

Scan for Video!

- **Objective:** Build endurance and strength in the lower body.
- **Focus:** Quads, glutes.
- **Position:** Stand with your back against the wall, feet about 2 feet from the wall.
- **Exercise:** Slide down the wall into a seated position, thighs parallel to the floor.
- **Breathing:** Maintain deep, steady breaths.

Time or Repetition:

- Beginner: Hold for 15 seconds.
- Intermediate: Hold for 30 seconds.
- Advanced: Hold for 45 seconds.

Cool Down: Slide back up to standing position.

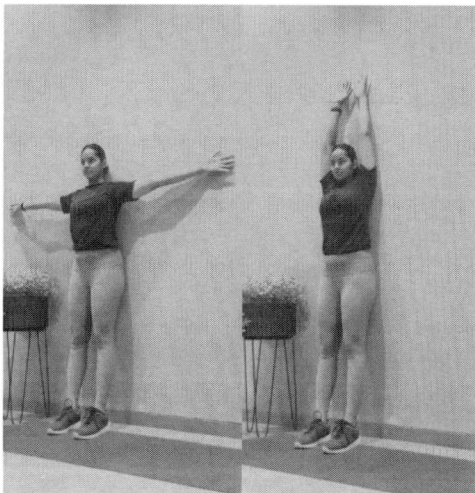

9. Wall Arm Slides

Scan for Video!

- **Objective:** Improve shoulder mobility and stretch the upper back.
- **Focus:** Shoulders, upper back.
- **Position:** Stand with your back to the wall, arms raised to shoulder height.
- **Exercise:** Slide your arms up the wall, keeping them as close to the wall as possible.
- **Breathing:** Inhale as arms go up, exhale as they return.

Time or Repetition:

- Beginner: 5 repetitions.
- Intermediate: 8 repetitions.
- Advanced: 10 repetitions.

Cool Down: Lower arms slowly, relax shoulders.

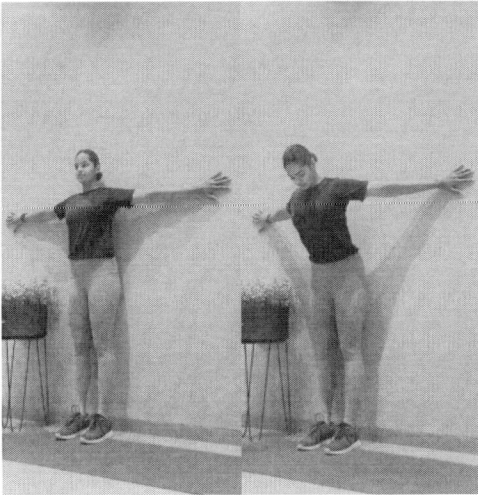

10. Wall Chest Opener

Scan for Video!

🎯 **Objective:** Stretch the chest and front shoulders, improving posture.

◎ **Focus:** Chest, shoulders.

⚓ **Position:** Stand facing away from the wall, arms extended out to the sides, palms on the wall.

💪 **Exercise:** Lean forward slightly, opening the chest.

🧘 **Breathing:** Deep inhales and exhales.

⏱ **Time or Repetition:**

- Beginner: Hold for 15 seconds.
- Intermediate: Hold for 20 seconds.
- Advanced: Hold for 25 seconds.

🧘 **Cool Down:** Release the stretch, shake out arms.

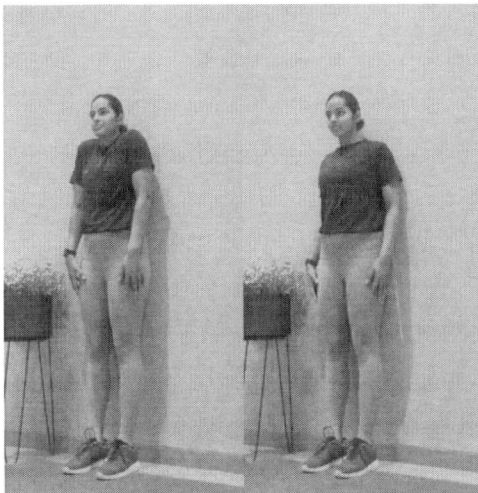

11. Wall Shoulder Rolls

Scan for Video!

🎯 **Objective:** Relieve tension in the shoulders and neck.

◎ **Focus:** Shoulders, neck.

⚓ **Position:** Stand with your back against the wall.

💪 **Exercise:** Roll your shoulders in a circular motion, up and back.

🧘 **Breathing:** Inhale up, exhale down.

⏱ **Time or Repetition:**

- Beginner: 5 rolls.
- Intermediate: 8 rolls.
- Advanced: 10 rolls.

🧘 **Cool Down:** Relax arms by your side, take deep breaths.

12. Wall Neck Extensions

Scan for Video!

- 🎯 **Objective:** Release tension in the neck and improve flexibility.

- ◎ **Focus:** Neck.

- ⚓ **Position:** Stand with your back against the wall, feet slightly forward.

- 💪 **Exercise:** Tilt your head back to touch the wall, then return to start.

- 🧘 **Breathing:** Inhale as you tilt back, exhale to return.

🕐 **Time or Repetition:**

- Beginner: 5 repetitions.

- Intermediate: 8 repetitions.

- Advanced: 10 repetitions.

🧘 **Cool Down:** Keep your head neutral, relax your neck muscles.

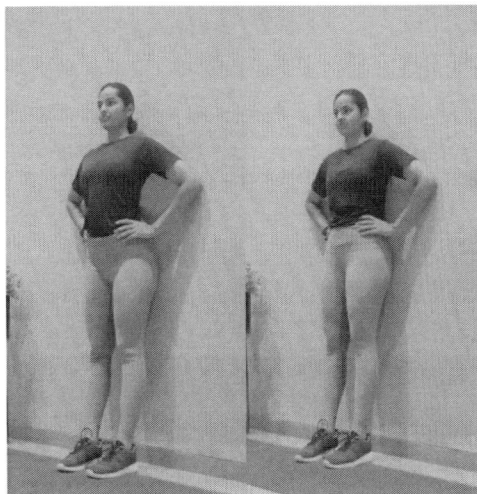

13. Wall Pelvic Tilt

Scan for Video!

- 🎯 **Objective:** Improve lower back and pelvic area flexibility, strengthen abdominal muscles.

- ◎ **Focus:** Lower back, abdominals, pelvis.

- ⚓ **Position:** Stand with your back against the wall, feet shoulder-width apart and slightly away from the wall.

- 💪 **Exercise:** Tilt your pelvis forward, flattening your lower back against the wall, then tilt it back to create a small arch.

- 🧘 **Breathing:** Inhale as you tilt forward, exhale as you return.

🕐 **Time or Repetition:**

- Beginner: 10 repetitions.

- Intermediate: 15 repetitions.

- Advanced: 20 repetitions.

🧘 **Cool Down:** Relax in a neutral standing position, deep breathing.

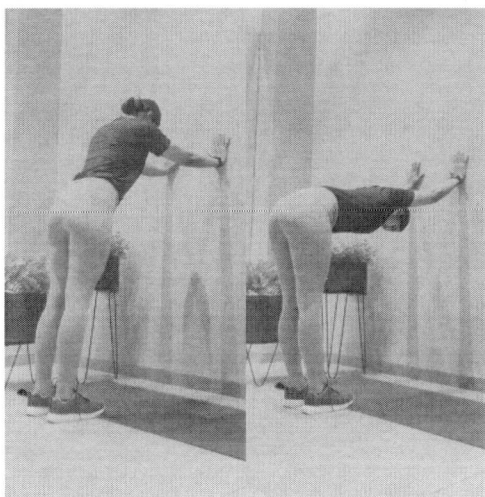

14. Wall Downward Dog

Scan for Video!

🎯 **Objective:** Stretch the shoulders, hamstrings, and calves; improve upper body strength.

◎ **Focus:** Shoulders, hamstrings, calves.

⚓ **Position:** Stand facing the wall, place hands on the wall at waist height, step back until your body forms a right angle.

🧘 **Exercise:** Press your chest toward the floor, feeling the stretch in your shoulders and back legs.

🧘 **Breathing:** Inhale as you lengthen the spine, exhale as you deepen the stretch.

⏱ **Time or Repetition:**

- Beginner: Hold for 15 seconds.
- Intermediate: Hold for 25 seconds.
- Advanced: Hold for 35 seconds.

🧘 **Cool Down:** Slowly walk towards the wall, rolling up to standing.

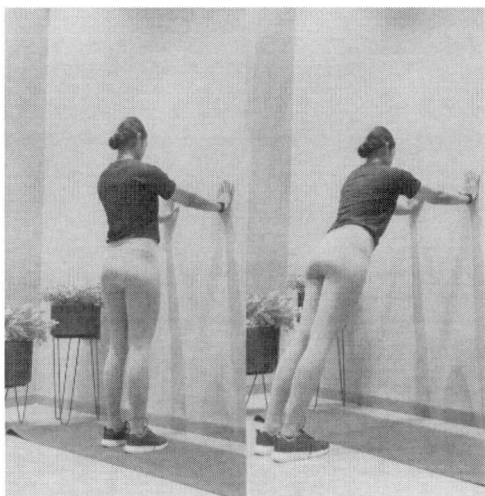

15. Wall Plank

Scan for Video!

🎯 **Objective:** Strengthen the core, shoulders, and arms.

◎ **Focus:** Core, shoulders, arms.

⚓ **Position:** Face the wall, extend arms to press palms against the wall, step back until body is in a plank position.

🧘 **Exercise:** Hold the plank with a straight line from head to heels.

🧘 **Breathing:** Maintain steady breathing.

⏱ **Time or Repetition:**

- Beginner: Hold for 20 seconds.
- Intermediate: Hold for 30 seconds.
- Advanced: Hold for 40 seconds.

🧘 **Cool Down:** Gradually step forward and relax.

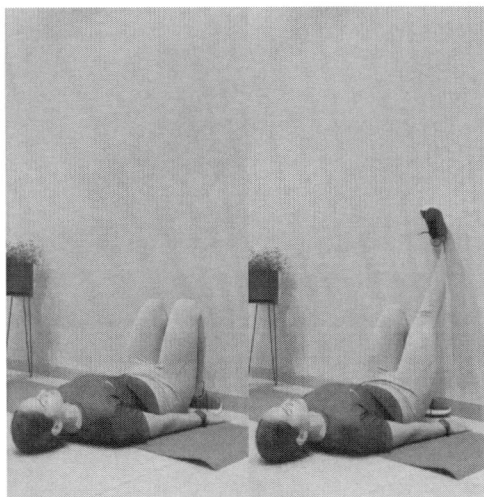

16. Wall Hamstring Stretch

Scan for Video!

🎯 **Objective:** Improve flexibility in the hamstrings and lower back.

◎ **Focus:** Hamstrings, lower back.

⚓ **Position:** Lie on your back a few inches from the wall, one leg extended up against the wall, the other flat on the ground.

💪 **Exercise:** Gently press the raised leg against the wall for a deep hamstring stretch.

🧍 **Breathing:** Inhale as you gently press, exhale as you release slightly.

🕐 **Time or Repetition:**

- Beginner: Hold for 20 seconds each leg.
- Intermediate: Hold for 30 seconds each leg.
- Advanced: Hold for 40 seconds each leg.

🧘 **Cool Down:** Slowly switch legs, then relax both legs on the floor.

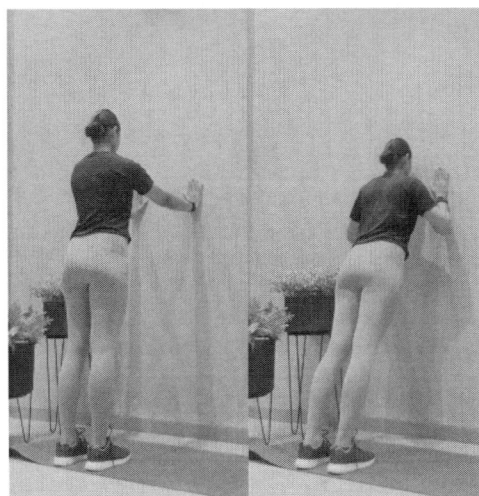

17. Wall Push-Up

Scan for Video!

🎯 **Objective:** Build strength in the chest, shoulders, and triceps.

◎ **Focus:** Chest, shoulders, triceps.

⚓ **Position:** Face the wall, place hands on the wall slightly wider than shoulder-width, step feet back.

💪 **Exercise:** Bend elbows to lower your body towards the wall, then push back.

🧍 **Breathing:** Inhale as you lower, exhale as you push back.

🕐 **Time or Repetition:**

- Beginner: 10 repetitions.
- Intermediate: 15 repetitions.
- Advanced: 20 repetitions.

🧘 **Cool Down:** Shake out the arms, deep breaths.

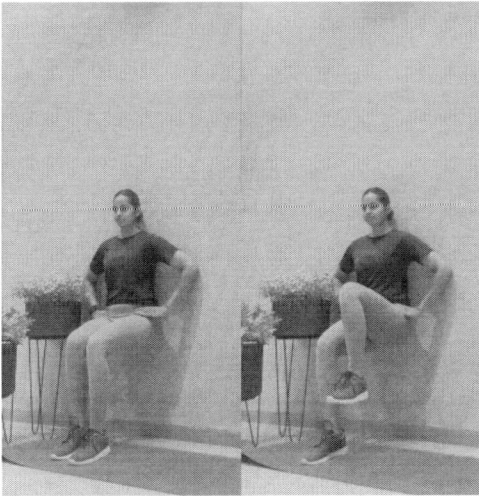

18. Wall Sit with Leg Raise

Scan for Video!

🎯 **Objective:** Strengthen the quadriceps, glutes, and core; improve balance.

◎ **Focus:** Quadriceps, glutes, core.

⚓ **Position:** Lean back against the wall in a sitting position, thighs parallel to the floor.

💪 **Exercise:** Alternate raising each leg while maintaining the wall sit position.

🧘 **Breathing:** Inhale as you raise a leg, exhale as you lower.

⏱ **Time or Repetition:**

- Beginner: 5 repetitions each leg.

- Intermediate: 8 repetitions each leg.

- Advanced: 10 repetitions each leg.

🧘 **Cool Down:** Slowly stand up, stretch the legs.

19. Wall Tree Pose

Scan for Video!

🎯 **Objective:** Improve balance and stability; strengthen the ankles, legs, and core.

◎ **Focus:** Balance, ankles, legs, core.

⚓ **Position:** Stand tall against the wall, weight on one foot, the other foot's sole against the inner thigh or calf (not the knee).

💪 **Exercise:** Press your foot against your leg, hands in prayer position or overhead.

🧘 **Breathing:** Maintain deep, steady breaths.

⏱ **Time or Repetition:**

- Beginner: Hold for 20 seconds each side.

- Intermediate: Hold for 30 seconds each side.

- Advanced: Hold for 40 seconds each side.

🧘 **Cool Down:** Gently release the pose, switch sides, then relax arms.

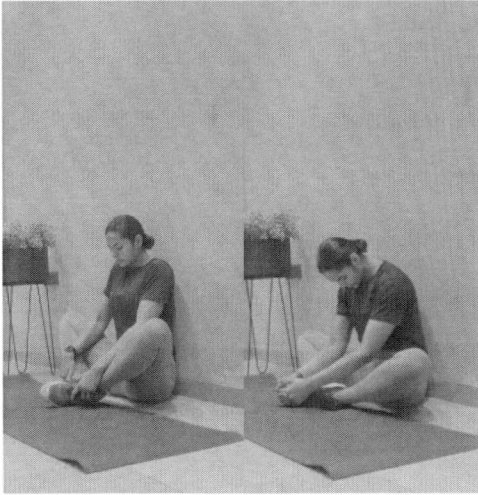

20. Wall Butterfly Stretch

Scan for Video!

🎯 **Objective:** Increase flexibility in the inner thighs, hips, and lower back.

◎ **Focus:** Inner thighs, hips, lower back.

⚓ **Position:** Sit with your back against the wall, soles of feet together, knees bent outwards.

💪 **Exercise:** Gently press knees towards the floor to deepen the stretch.

🧘 **Breathing:** Inhale as you sit up tall, exhale as you press the knees down.

⏱ **Time or Repetition:**

- Beginner: Hold for 20 seconds.

- Intermediate: Hold for 30 seconds.

- Advanced: Hold for 40 seconds.

🧘 **Cool Down:** Carefully release the legs, straighten them out, and shake gently.

21. Wall Palms Slide

Scan for Video!

🎯 **Objective:** Increase shoulder mobility and stretch the upper back.

◎ **Focus:** Shoulders, upper back.

⚓ **Position:** Stand facing the wall, arms extended with palms flat against the wall at shoulder height.

💪 **Exercise:** Slowly slide palms up the wall as high as possible without straining, then slide them back down.

🧘 **Breathing:** Inhale as you slide up, exhale as you return.

⏱ **Time or Repetition:**
- Beginner: 5 repetitions.

- Intermediate: 8 repetitions.

- Advanced: 10 repetitions.

🧘 **Cool Down:** Relax arms by your side and roll shoulders gently.

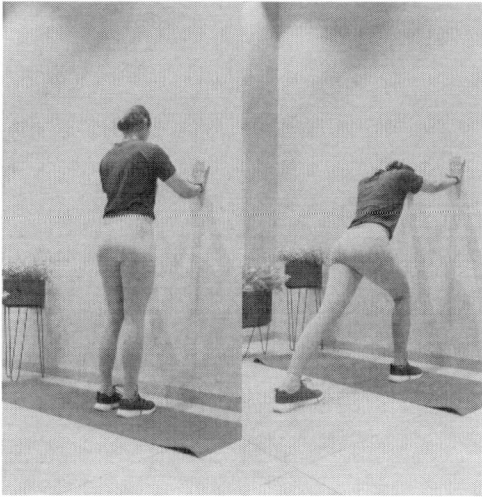

22. Wall Supported Ankle Stretches

Scan for Video!

- **Objective:** Improve ankle flexibility and mobility.

- **Focus:** Ankles, calves.

- **Position:** Stand arm's length from the wall, hands on the wall for support.

- **Exercise:** Extend one leg back, keeping the heel down and toes pointed towards the wall, to stretch the ankle and calf.

- **Breathing:** Inhale as you press the heel down, exhale as you ease off.

Time or Repetition:

- Beginner: Hold for 20 seconds each ankle.

- Intermediate: Hold for 30 seconds each ankle.

- Advanced: Hold for 40 seconds each ankle.

Cool Down: Gently shake out each leg after stretching.

23. Wall Assisted Knee Lifts

Scan for Video!

- **Objective:** Strengthen lower abdominals and improve hip mobility.

- **Focus:** Lower abdominals, hips.

- **Position:** Stand with your back to the wall, feet hip-width apart.

- **Exercise:** Lift one knee towards the chest, then lower it, alternating legs.

- **Breathing:** Inhale as you lift the knee, exhale as you lower.

Time or Repetition:

- Beginner: 10 repetitions each leg.

- Intermediate: 15 repetitions each leg.

- Advanced: 20 repetitions each leg.

Cool Down: Stand still, deep breathing.

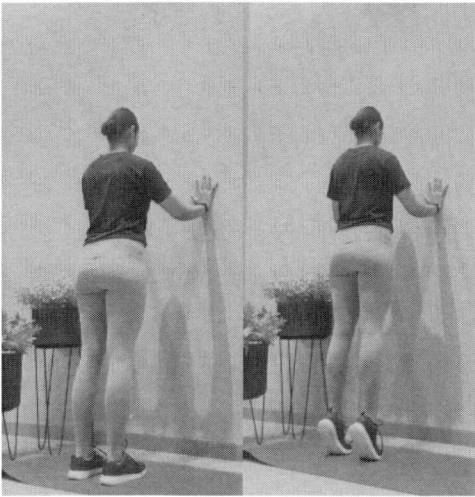

24. Wall Assisted Calf Raises

Scan for Video!

🎯 **Objective:** Strengthen calf muscles and improve ankle stability.

◎ **Focus:** Calves, ankles.

⚓ **Position:** Face the wall, hands on the wall for support, feet hip-width apart.

💪 **Exercise:** Raise heels off the ground as high as possible, then lower.

🧘 **Breathing:** Inhale as you raise, exhale as you lower.

⏱ **Time or Repetition:**

- Beginner: 10 repetitions.
- Intermediate: 15 repetitions.
- Advanced: 20 repetitions.

🧘 **Cool Down:** Roll feet gently on the ground.

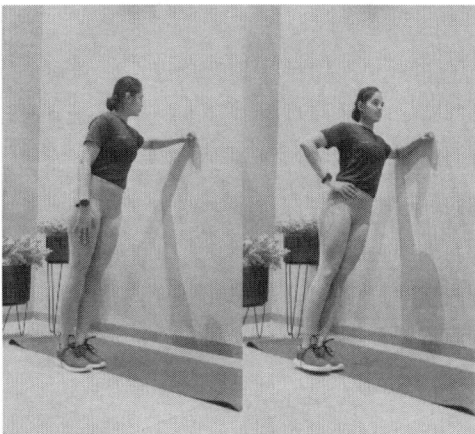

25. Wall Supported Side Plank

Scan for Video!

🎯 **Objective:** Enhance core and side muscles' strength, improve balance.

◎ **Focus:** Core, obliques, shoulders.

⚓ **Position:** Lie on your side, feet against the wall, elbow under shoulder, and lift your hips to create a straight line.

💪 **Exercise:** Hold the side plank position, pushing feet against the wall for stability.

🧘 **Breathing:** Maintain steady breathing.

⏱ **Time or Repetition:**

- Beginner: Hold for 15 seconds each side.
- Intermediate: Hold for 25 seconds each side.
- Advanced: Hold for 35 seconds each side.

🧘 **Cool Down:** Gently lower your hips, switch sides, and repeat.

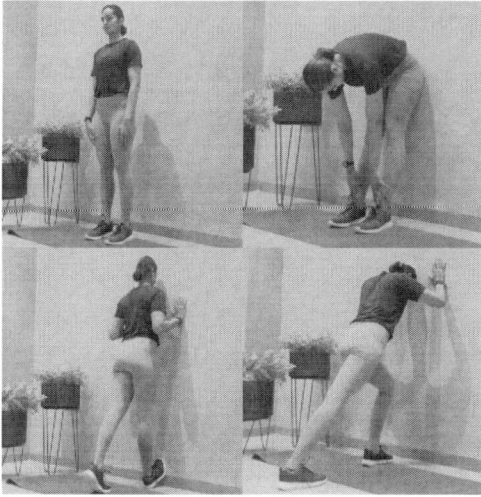

26. Wall Supported Flexibility Routine

Scan for Video!

- 🎯 **Objective:** Improve overall flexibility through a series of wall-supported stretches.
- ◎ **Focus:** Full body.
- ⚓ **Position:** Use the wall for support in various stretching positions, such as hamstring stretch, side stretches, and calf stretches.
- 💪 **Exercise:** Perform a series of stretches with the wall's aid to target different body parts.

🧘 **Breathing:** Inhale into each stretch, exhale as you deepen the stretch.

⏱ **Time or Repetition:**

- Beginner: Hold each stretch for 20 seconds.
- Intermediate: Hold each stretch for 30 seconds.
- Advanced: Hold each stretch for 40 seconds.

🧘 **Cool Down:** Slow, deep breathing as you gently release from each stretch.

27. Wall Supported Relaxation

Scan for Video!

- 🎯 **Objective:** Promote relaxation and reduce stress through supported wall poses.
- ◎ **Focus:** Relaxation, stress reduction.
- ⚓ **Position:** Sit or lie comfortably close to or against the wall in a relaxed posture.
- 💪 **Exercise:** Use the wall to support your body in a comfortable position that allows for relaxation, such as legs up the wall.
- 🧘 **Breathing:** Deep, slow breaths to promote relaxation.

⏱ **Time or Repetition:**

- Beginner: 5 minutes.
- Intermediate: 7 minutes.
- Advanced: 10 minutes.

🧘 **Cool Down:** Slowly transition to a seated position, taking a moment to enjoy the calmness.

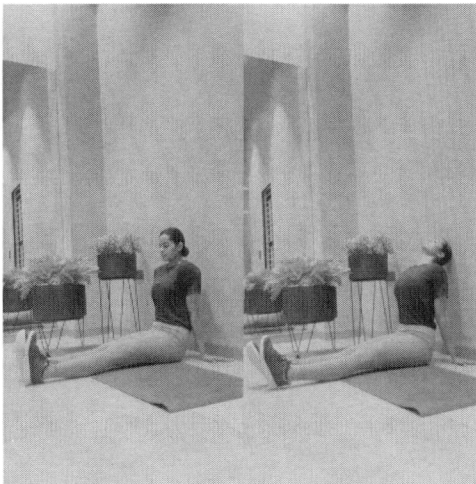

28. Wall Supported Fish Pose

Scan for Video!

🎯 **Objective:** Open the chest and shoulders, improve respiratory function.

◎ **Focus:** Chest, shoulders, thoracic spine.

⚓ **Position:** Sit with your back against the wall, legs extended forward, hands on the floor behind you, fingers pointing away.

🏋 **Exercise:** Press into your hands to lift the chest towards the ceiling, gently tilting the head back if comfortable.

🧘 **Breathing:** Deep inhales as you open the chest, exhales as you gently release.

🕐 **Time or Repetition:**

- Beginner: Hold for 20 seconds.

- Intermediate: Hold for 30 seconds.

- Advanced: Hold for 40 seconds.

🧘 **Cool Down:** Gently release the pose, sitting tall against the wall, taking deep breaths.

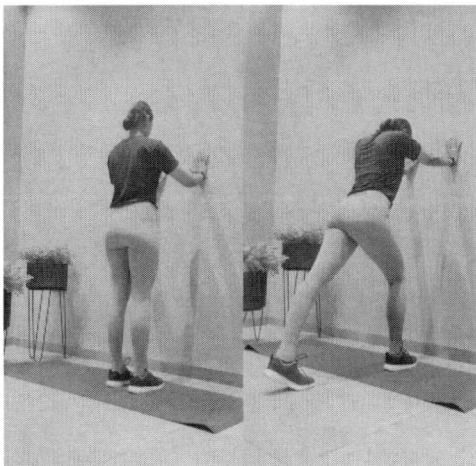

29. Wall Supported Hamstring stretch

Scan for Video!

🎯 **Objective:** Release tension in the back and legs, and promote relaxation.

◎ **Focus:** Back, shoulders, legs.

⚓ **Position:** Stand in front of the wall, arms extended with hands on the wall, one leg extended behind, on your toes.

🏋 **Exercise:** Press your hands into the wall and try to straighten your back leg as much as possible, aiming to deepen the stretch in your shoulders.

🧘 **Breathing:** Deep inhales and exhales, focusing on relaxing your body with each exhale.

🕐 **Time or Repetition:**

- Beginner: Hold for 30 seconds.

- Intermediate: Hold for 45 seconds.

- Advanced: Hold for 60 seconds.

🧘 **Cool Down:** Slowly stand, and relax your shoulders.

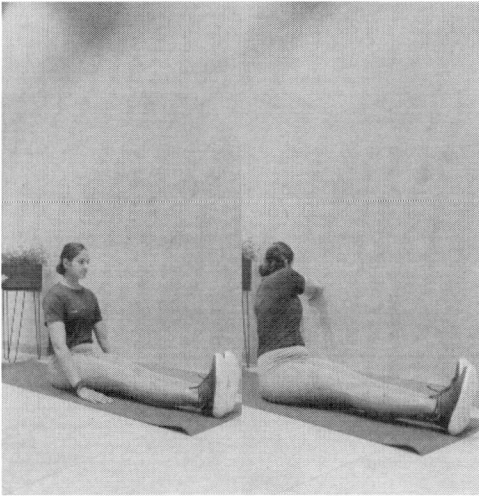

30. Wall Supported Spinal Twist

Scan for Video!

◎ **Objective:** Improve spinal mobility and release tension in the lower back.

◎ **Focus:** Spine, lower back.

⚓ **Position:** Sit sideways next to the wall, legs extended in front of you. Rotate your torso to place your hands on the wall behind you.

🏋 **Exercise:** Gently press into the wall to deepen the twist, turning your head to look over your shoulder if comfortable.

🧘 **Breathing:** Inhale as you lengthen the spine, exhale as you deepen the twist.

⏱ **Time or Repetition:**

- Beginner: Hold for 20 seconds each side.

- Intermediate: Hold for 30 seconds each side.

- Advanced: Hold for 40 seconds each side.

🧘 **Cool Down:** Return to center, switch sides, then relax.

31. Wall Supported Shoulder Stand

Scan for Video!

◎ **Objective:** Strengthen the shoulders, neck, and spine; improve circulation.

◎ **Focus:** Shoulders, neck, spine.

⚓ **Position:** Lie on your back with your legs up the wall, arms on the floor for support.

🏋 **Exercise:** Lift your hips off the floor, using your hands to support your lower back. Aim to straighten the legs vertically.

🧘 **Breathing:** Steady breathing, focusing on stability.

⏱ **Time or Repetition:**

- Beginner: Hold for 20 seconds.

- Intermediate: Hold for 30 seconds.

- Advanced: Hold for 40 seconds.

🧘 **Cool Down:** Slowly lower your hips back to the floor, legs down.

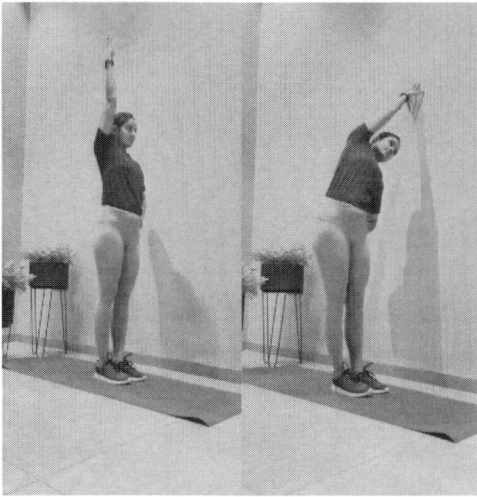

3.2 – For Intermediate

32. Wall Triangle Pose

Scan for Video!

🎯 **Objective:** Stretch the sides of the body, improve flexibility in the legs, and strengthen the core.

◎ **Focus:** Sides of the body, legs, core.

⚓ **Position:** Stand perpendicular to the wall, feet wide apart, extend one arm up and place the other on the wall.

💪 **Exercise:** Reach the top arm over your head towards the wall, creating a deep side stretch while both legs remain straight.

🧘 **Breathing:** Inhale as you extend, exhale as you deepen the stretch.

⏱ **Time or Repetition:**

- Beginner: Hold for 20 seconds each side.

- Intermediate: Hold for 30 seconds each side.

- Advanced: Hold for 40 seconds each side.

🧘 **Cool Down:** Return to starting position, switch sides.

33. Wall Warrior Pose

Scan for Video!

🎯 **Objective:** Increase lower body strength, improve balance and stability.

◎ **Focus:** Legs, core, balance.

⚓ **Position:** Stand facing the wall, one foot forward and one back, bending the front knee, hands on the wall.

💪 **Exercise:** Press into the wall while maintaining a strong warrior pose, back leg straight, front knee bent.

🧘 **Breathing:** Inhale and exhale steadily, focusing on maintaining balance and strength.

⏱ **Time or Repetition:**

- Beginner: Hold for 20 seconds each side.

- Intermediate: Hold for 30 seconds each side.

- Advanced: Hold for 40 seconds each side.

🧘 **Cool Down:** Straighten the front leg, switch sides.

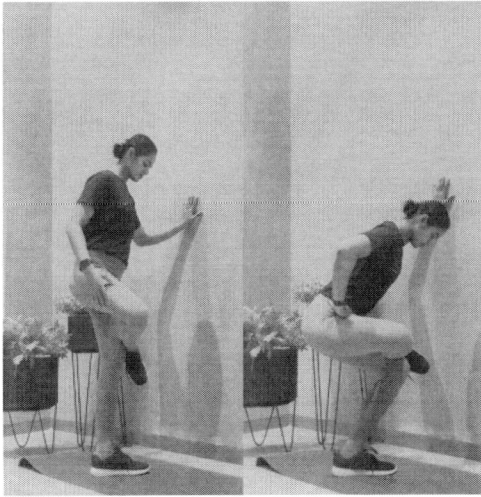

34. Wall Pigeon Pose

Scan for Video!

🎯 **Objective:** Open the hips and stretch the thighs, glutes, and lower back.

◎ **Focus:** Hips, thighs, glutes, lower back.

⚓ **Position:** Stand facing the wall, place one leg up with the shin against the wall, and slide the other leg back.

💪 **Exercise:** Lower your body towards the floor or a comfortable depth to stretch the hip of the front leg.

🧘 **Breathing:** Deep inhales and exhales, relaxing into the stretch.

⏱ **Time or Repetition:**

- Beginner: Hold for 30 seconds each side.

- Intermediate: Hold for 45 seconds each side.

- Advanced: Hold for 60 seconds each side.

🧘 **Cool Down:** Gently release the pose, switch legs.

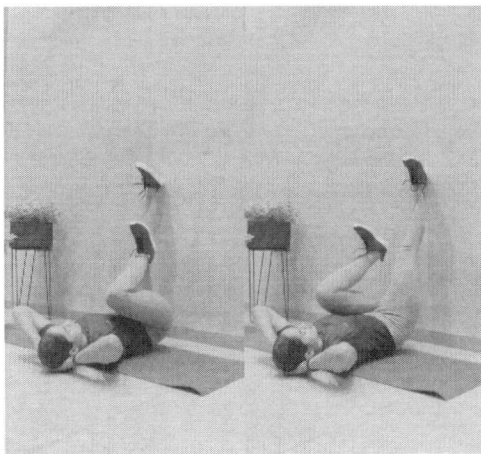

35. Wall Supported Bicycle

Scan for Video!

🎯 **Objective:** Enhance core strength and leg mobility.

◎ **Focus:** Core, legs.

⚓ **Position:** Lie on your back with your legs up and press against the wall, hands behind your head.

💪 **Exercise:** Alternate bending and straightening legs in a cycling motion, pressing the back flat against the floor.

🧘 **Breathing:** Inhale as one leg bends, exhale as it straightens.

⏱ **Time or Repetition:**

- Beginner: 30 seconds.

- Intermediate: 45 seconds.

- Advanced: 60 seconds.

🧘 **Cool Down:** Rest legs against the wall, deep breathing.

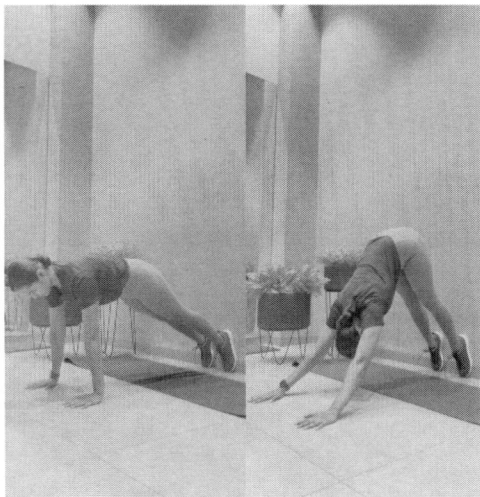

36. Wall Supported Downward Facing Dog

Scan for Video!

🎯 **Objective:** Strengthen the arms and shoulders, stretch the spine and legs.

◎ **Focus:** Arms, shoulders, spine, legs.

⚓ **Position:** Stand facing away from the wall, hands on the floor in a pike position, feet back, heels up.

🤸 **Exercise:** Walk your feet up the wall to a comfortable height, pushing the floor away to deepen the stretch.

🧘 **Breathing:** Inhale as you lengthen the spine, exhale as you press heels towards the wall.

⏱ **Time or Repetition:**

- Beginner: Hold for 20 seconds.
- Intermediate: Hold for 30 seconds.
- Advanced: Hold for 40 seconds.

🧘 **Cool Down:** Walk feet down, return to standing slowly.

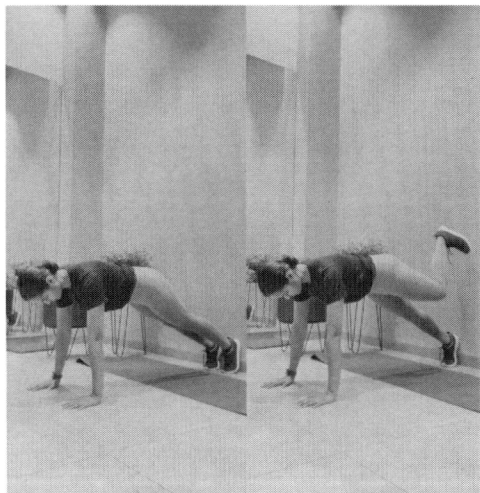

37. Wall Supported Plank with Leg Raise

Scan for Video!

🎯 **Objective:** Strengthen the core and increase lower body control.

◎ **Focus:** Core, glutes, lower back.

⚓ **Position:** Face the wall in a plank position, hands on the ground, feet against the wall.

🤸 **Exercise:** Alternate raising each leg off the wall while maintaining a strong plank position.

🧘 **Breathing:** Inhale as one leg raises, exhale as it lowers.

⏱ **Time or Repetition:**

- Beginner: 5 repetitions each leg.
- Intermediate: 8 repetitions each leg.
- Advanced: 10 repetitions each leg.

🧘 **Cool Down:** Lower knees to the floor, relax in child's pose.

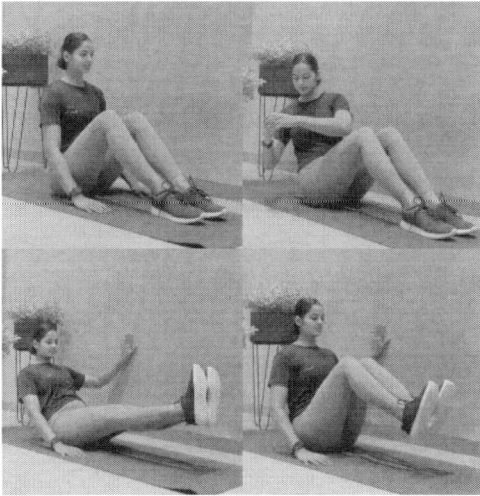

38. Wall Supported Core Workout

Scan for Video!

🎯 **Objective:** Enhance core stability and strength through various exercises.

◎ **Focus:** Core, abdominals.

⚓ **Position:** Various positions utilizing the wall for support, such as planks, leg raises, and twists.

💪 **Exercise:** Perform a series of core-focused exercises with the wall providing support and resistance.

🧘 **Breathing:** Coordinate breath with movement, focusing on exhaling during the effort phase.

⏱ **Time or Repetition:**

- Beginner: 30 seconds per exercise.

- Intermediate: 45 seconds per exercise.

- Advanced: 60 seconds per exercise.

🧘 **Cool Down:** Gentle stretching of the abdominal muscles and deep breathing.

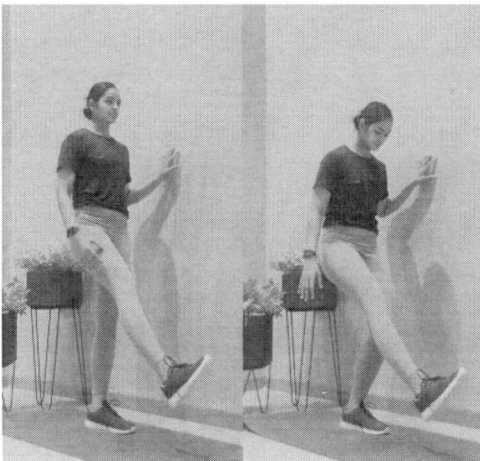

39. Wall Supported Balance Challenge

Scan for Video!

🎯 **Objective:** Improve balance and proprioception, strengthen stabilizing muscles.

◎ **Focus:** Balance, core, lower body.

⚓ **Position:** Stand on one leg close to the wall, using the wall lightly for balance if needed.

💪 **Exercise:** Maintain balance on one leg, try various arm positions or slight squats to challenge stability.

🧘 **Breathing:** Steady breaths, focusing on a fixed point to aid balance.

⏱ **Time or Repetition:**

- Beginner: Hold for 20 seconds each leg.

- Intermediate: Hold for 30 seconds each leg.

- Advanced: Hold for 40 seconds each leg, adding movements.

🧘 **Cool Down:** Shake out the legs, deep breathing.

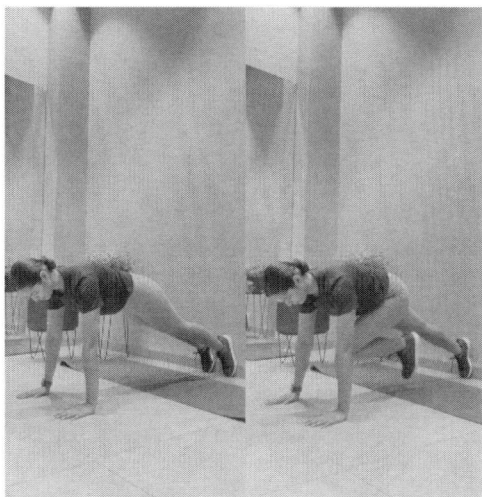

40. Wall Mountain Climbers

Scan for Video!

🎯 **Objective:** Boost cardiovascular health, strengthen the core, and improve agility.

◎ **Focus:** Cardiovascular system, core, arms, legs.

⚓ **Position:** Start in a plank position with feet against the wall.

💪 **Exercise:** Quickly alternate driving knees towards the chest, mimicking the mountain climber movement.

🧘 **Breathing:** Rapid breaths, inhale and exhale with each knee drive.

⏱ **Time or Repetition:**

- Beginner: 30 seconds.

- Intermediate: 45 seconds.

- Advanced: 60 seconds.

🧘 **Cool Down:** Slowly lower to knees, rest in a seated position, deep breathing.

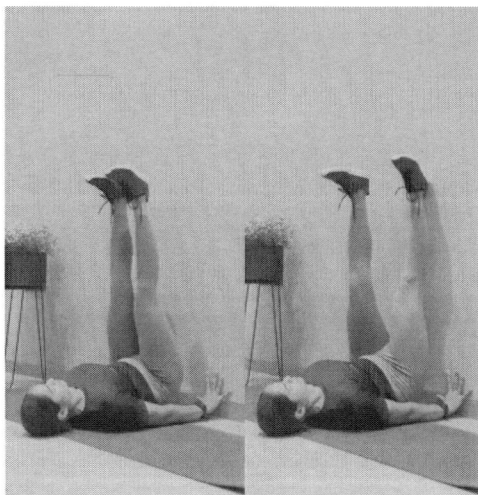

41. Wall Scissor Kicks

Scan for Video!

🎯 **Objective:** Enhance lower abdominal strength and improve hip flexor flexibility.

◎ **Focus:** Lower abdominals, hip flexors.

⚓ **Position:** Lie on your back with your buttocks close to the wall, legs straight up against the wall.

💪 **Exercise:** Lower one leg down towards the floor while keeping the other vertical, alternate in a scissor motion.

🧘 **Breathing:** Inhale as one leg moves down, exhale as it comes up.

⏱ **Time or Repetition:**

- Beginner: 30 seconds.

- Intermediate: 45 seconds.

- Advanced: 60 seconds.

🧘 **Cool Down:** Gently hug knees to chest, rocking side to side.

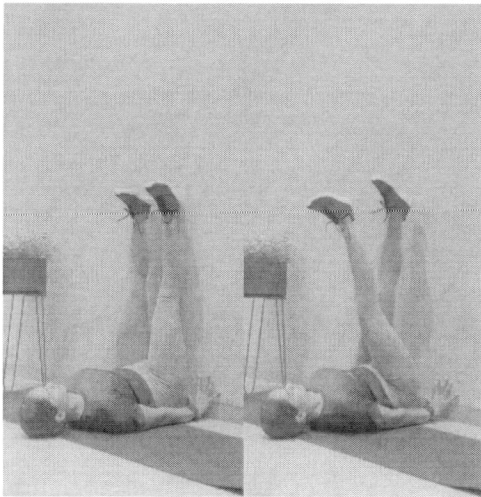

42. Wall Flutter Kicks

Scan for Video!

🎯 **Objective:** Strengthen the core and lower back, increase endurance in lower abdominals.

◎ **Focus:** Core, lower back, abdominals.

⚓ **Position:** Lie on your back with your buttocks close to the wall, legs extended straight up against the wall.

💪 **Exercise:** Perform small, rapid vertical movements with each leg, alternating in a flutter motion.

🧘 **Breathing:** Steady breathing, focus on exhaling during more challenging parts of the exercise.

⏱ **Time or Repetition:**

- Beginner: 30 seconds.
- Intermediate: 45 seconds.
- Advanced: 60 seconds.

🧘 **Cool Down:** Rest legs against the wall, deep breathing to relax.

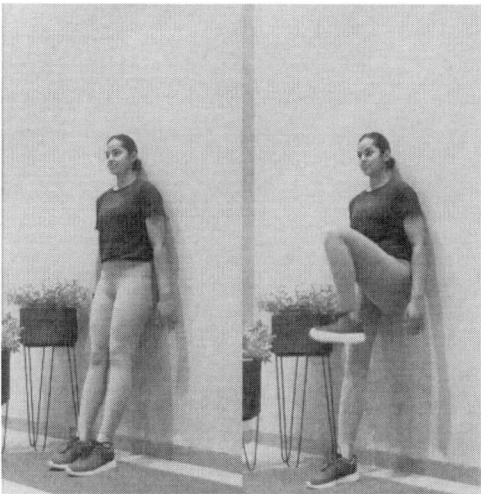

43. Wall Marching

Scan for Video!

🎯 **Objective:** Improve lower body coordination, strengthen the core, and enhance stability.

◎ **Focus:** Core, hip flexors, legs.

⚓ **Position:** Stand with your back against the wall, feet hip-width apart.

💪 **Exercise:** Alternate lifting knees as if marching in place, keeping the back flat against the wall.

🧘 **Breathing:** Inhale as you lift one knee, exhale as you lower.

⏱ **Time or Repetition:**

- Beginner: 1 minute.
- Intermediate: 2 minutes.
- Advanced: 3 minutes.

🧘 **Cool Down:** Stand still, deep breathing to relax.

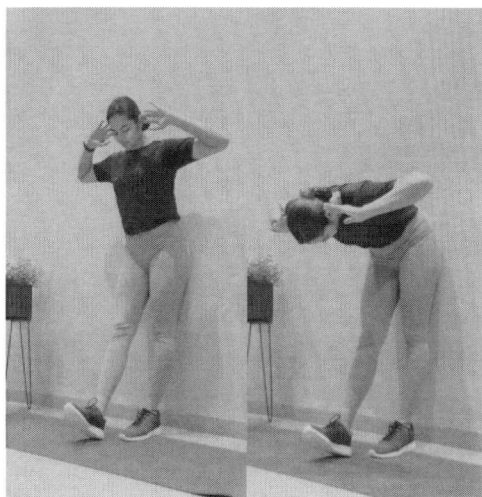

44. Balance hamstring stretch

Scan for Video!

🎯 **Objective:** Stretches hamstrings, strengthens lower back, improves concentration and balance.

◎ **Focus:** Legs, hips, concentration.

⚓ **Position:** Stand slightly facing away from the wall, feet under hips, one foot one step ahead, hands behind the ears, elbows flared out.

💪 **Exercise:** Lean forward from the lower back, without arching the back as much as possible.

🧘 **Breathing:** Deep breaths, focusing on maintaining balance and form.

⏱ **Time or Repetition:**

- Beginner: Hold for 20 seconds each side.

- Intermediate: Hold for 30 seconds each side.

- Advanced: Hold for 40 seconds each side.

🧎 **Cool Down:** Gently straighten the front leg, switch sides, then relax arms by sides.

45. Wall Supported Squat Slide

Scan for Video!

🎯 **Objective:** Build strength in the lower body, improve squat form.

◎ **Focus:** Quads, glutes, hamstrings.

⚓ **Position:** Stand with your back against the wall, feet shoulder-width apart.

💪 **Exercise:** Slide down the wall into a squat position, thighs parallel to the floor, then slide back up.

🧘 **Breathing:** Inhale as you slide down, exhale as you return to standing.

⏱ **Time or Repetition:**

- Beginner: 10 repetitions.

- Intermediate: 15 repetitions.

- Advanced: 20 repetitions.

🧎 **Cool Down:** Stand tall, stretch legs individually.

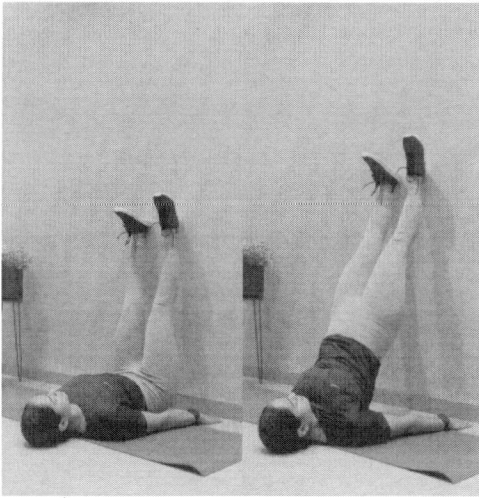

46. Wall Roll Over

Scan for Video!

🎯 **Objective:** Enhance spine flexibility, strengthen abdominals.

◎ **Focus:** Spine, abdominals.

⚓ **Position:** Lie on your back with legs extended up the wall.

💪 **Exercise:** Use abdominal muscles to lift hips off the floor, rolling towards the wall, then slowly roll down.

🧘 **Breathing:** Exhale as you roll up, inhale as you return.

⏱ **Time or Repetition:**

- Beginner: 5 repetitions.

- Intermediate: 8 repetitions.

- Advanced: 10 repetitions.

🧘 **Cool Down:** Rest legs up the wall, deep breathing.

47. Wall Standing Leg Extension

Scan for Video!

🎯 **Objective:** Strengthen quadriceps and improve balance.

◎ **Focus:** Quadriceps, balance.

⚓ **Position:** Stand facing the wall, hands on the wall for balance.

💪 **Exercise:** Lift one leg at a time, extending it straight back, keeping the hip squared.

🧘 **Breathing:** Inhale as you lift, exhale as you extend.

⏱ **Time or Repetition:**

- Beginner: 10 repetitions each leg.

- Intermediate: 15 repetitions each leg.

- Advanced: 20 repetitions each leg.

🧘 **Cool Down:** Gently shake legs, stand tall.

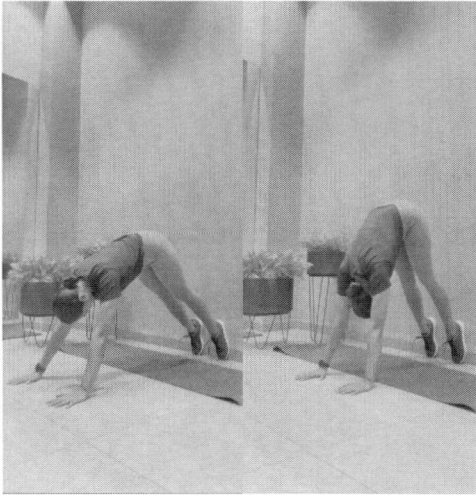

48. Wall Pike

Scan for Video!

🎯 **Objective:** Increase shoulder strength and flexibility, improve core stability.

◎ **Focus:** Shoulders, core, hamstrings.

⚓ **Position:** Start in a downward dog position with feet against the wall.

💪 **Exercise:** Walk feet up the wall to a comfortable height, aiming to form an inverted "V" with the body.

🧘 **Breathing:** Steady breaths, focusing on form.

⏱ **Time or Repetition:**

- Beginner: Hold for 15 seconds.

- Intermediate: Hold for 25 seconds.

- Advanced: Hold for 35 seconds.

🧘 **Cool Down:** Walk feet down the wall, rest in child's pose.

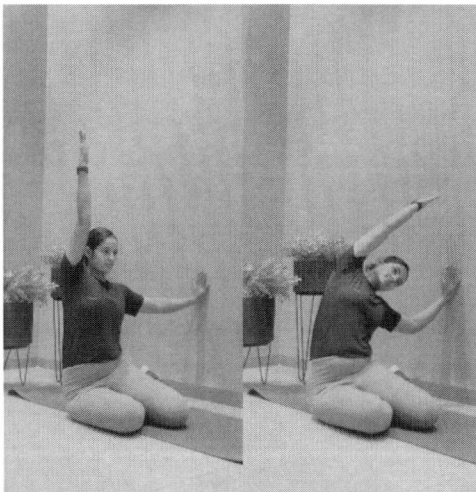

49. Wall Mermaid Pose

Scan for Video!

🎯 **Objective:** Open up the side body, stretch the shoulders and hips.

◎ **Focus:** Side body, shoulders, hips.

⚓ **Position:** Sit with one hip close to the wall, legs folded to one side, one hand on the wall.

💪 **Exercise:** Reach the other arm overhead towards the wall, creating a side stretch.

🧘 **Breathing:** Inhale to lengthen, exhale to deepen the stretch.

⏱ **Time or Repetition:**

- Beginner: Hold for 20 seconds each side.

- Intermediate: Hold for 30 seconds each side.

- Advanced: Hold for 40 seconds each side.

🧘 **Cool Down:** Gently release, switch sides.

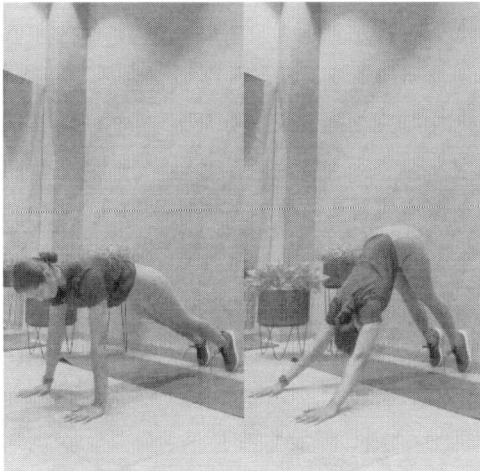

50. Wall Pike Slides

Scan for Video!

- ⊙ **Objective:** Enhance core strength, improve flexibility in hamstrings and lower back.

- ⊙ **Focus:** Core, hamstrings, lower back.

- ⚓ **Position:** Start in a downward dog position with feet against the wall.

- 💪 **Exercise:** Slide feet up the wall into a pike position, then slide back down.

- 🧘 **Breathing:** Inhale as you slide up, exhale as you return.

⏱ **Time or Repetition:**

- Beginner: 5 repetitions.

- Intermediate: 8 repetitions.

- Advanced: 10 repetitions.

🧘 **Cool Down:** Rest in child's pose, deep breathing.

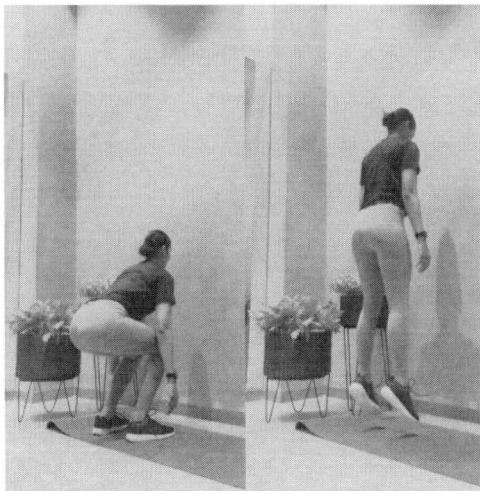

51. Wall Jump Squats

Scan for Video!

- ⊙ **Objective:** Build explosive leg strength, increase heart rate for cardiovascular benefits.

- ⊙ **Focus:** Quads, glutes, cardiovascular system.

- ⚓ **Position:** Stand with your back against the wall, feet shoulder-width apart.

- 💪 **Exercise:** Perform a squat, then explosively jump upwards, landing softly in a squat.

- 🧘 **Breathing:** Inhale to squat, exhale to jump.

⏱ **Time or Repetition:**

- Beginner: 10 repetitions.

- Intermediate: 15 repetitions.

- Advanced: 20 repetitions.

🧘 **Cool Down:** Stand tall, deep breaths, stretch legs.

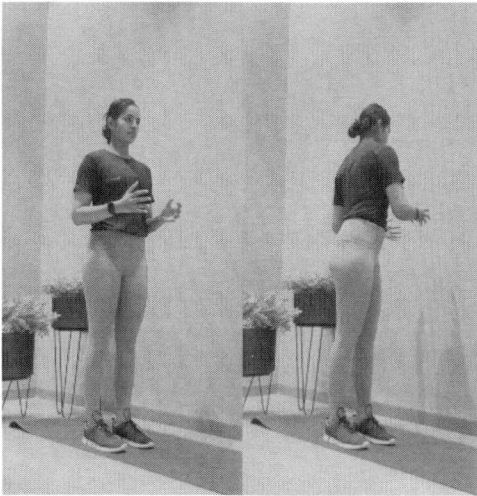

52. Wall Oblique Twists

Scan for Video!

◎ **Objective:** Strengthen the oblique muscles, improve rotational mobility.

◎ **Focus:** Obliques, core.

⚓ **Position:** Stand side-on to the wall, a step away, holding a lightweight object or none.

💪 **Exercise:** Rotate the torso to gently toss the object against the wall, catch it, and twist to the other side.

🧘 **Breathing:** Inhale as you twist, exhale as you release.

⏱ **Time or Repetition:**

- Beginner: 1 minute.
- Intermediate: 2 minutes.
- Advanced: 3 minutes.

🧘 **Cool Down:** Stand tall, hands on hips, gently twist torso side to side.

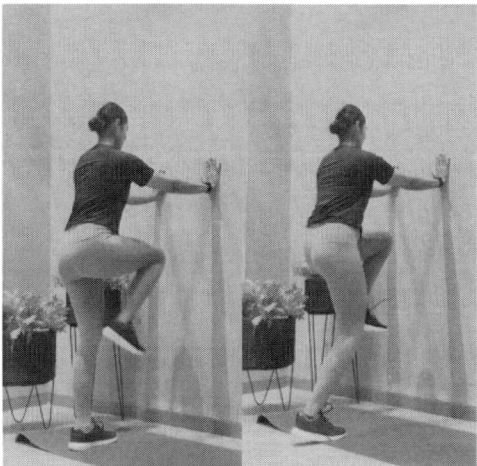

53. Wall High Knees

Scan for Video!

◎ **Objective:** Improve cardiovascular fitness, strengthen lower body.

◎ **Focus:** Cardiovascular system, quads, hip flexors.

⚓ **Position:** Face the wall, lightly touching it for balance.

💪 **Exercise:** Run in place, bringing knees up high towards the chest.

🧘 **Breathing:** Quick breaths, in rhythm with knee lifts.

⏱ **Time or Repetition:**

- Beginner: 30 seconds.
- Intermediate: 45 seconds.
- Advanced: 60 seconds.

🧘 **Cool Down:** Slow march in place, deep breathing.

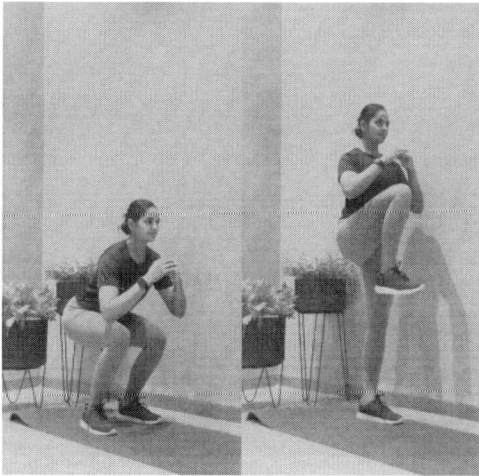

54. Wall Tuck Jumps

Scan for Video!

🎯 **Objective:** Build lower body power and improve cardiovascular health.

◎ **Focus:** Quads, glutes, cardiovascular system.

⚓ **Position:** Stand a small distance from the wall, feet hip-width apart.

💪 **Exercise:** Perform a squat, then explosively jump upwards, tucking knees towards the chest.

🧘 **Breathing:** Inhale to squat, exhale on the jump.

⏱ **Time or Repetition:**

- Beginner: 5 repetitions.
- Intermediate: 8 repetitions.
- Advanced: 10 repetitions.

🧎 **Cool Down:** Gentle jog in place, then stretch.

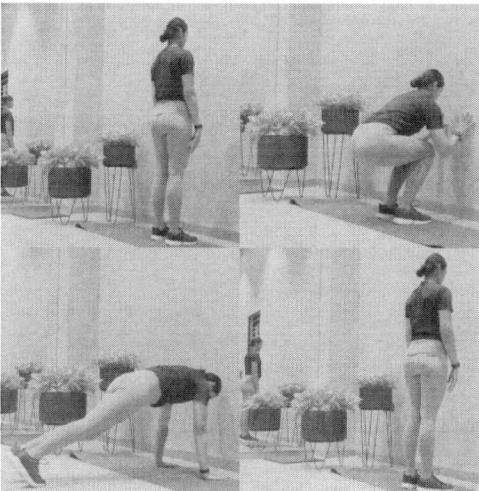

55. Wall Burpees

Scan for Video!

🎯 **Objective:** Increase full-body strength, endurance, and agility.

◎ **Focus:** Full body, cardiovascular endurance.

⚓ **Position:** Stand facing the wall, a couple of feet away.

💪 **Exercise:** Perform a standard burpee with a push-up at the bottom, then jump up to touch the wall.

🧘 **Breathing:** Inhale on the way down, exhale during the push-up and jump.

⏱ **Time or Repetition:**

- Beginner: 5 repetitions.
- Intermediate: 8 repetitions.
- Advanced: 10 repetitions.

🧎 **Cool Down:** Walk in place, gradually slowing down, then stretch.

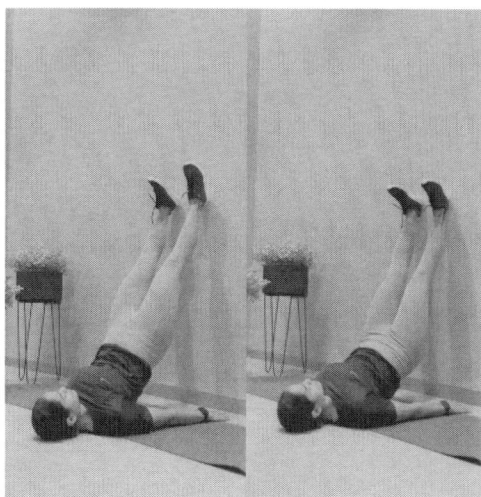

56. Wall-Supported Bridge Lift

Scan for Video!

- **Objective:** Strengthen the core and lower back, improve leg strength and flexibility, offering similar benefits to the Wall Supported Shoulder Stand but with focus on lower body engagement.
- **Focus:** Core, lower back, glutes, hamstrings.
- **Position:** Lie on your back with your feet extended upwards against the wall, knees straight, and arms by your sides for support.
- **Exercise:** Press your feet into the wall to lift your hips towards the ceiling, creating a straightened bridge. Ensure your shoulders and arms remain flat on the ground for stability.

Breathing: Inhale as you prepare, exhale as you lift your hips upwards.

Time or Repetition:

- Beginner: Hold for 15 seconds, 5 repetitions.
- Intermediate: Hold for 20 seconds, 8 repetitions.
- Advanced: Hold for 25 seconds, 10 repetitions.

Cool Down: Gently lower your hips to the floor, hug your knees to your chest, and rock gently side to side to relax the spine.

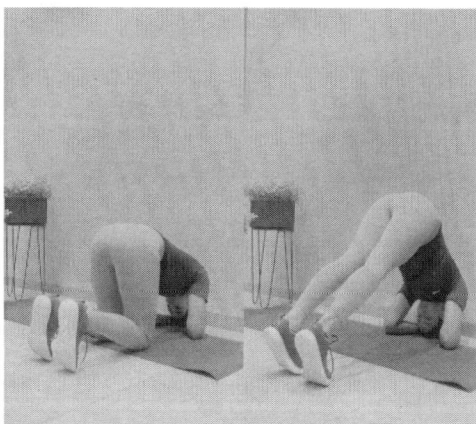

57. Wall Supported Headstand

Scan for Video!

- **Objective:** Build upper body and core strength, improve balance, and increase blood flow to the brain.
- **Focus:** Arms, core, balance.
- **Position:** Kneel facing away from the wall, place your forearms on the ground, interlace your fingers, and place the top of your head on the floor between your hands.
- **Exercise:** Walk your feet up the wall until your body is in a straight line, keeping your core engaged.

Breathing: Breathe deeply, focusing on maintaining a steady and controlled breath.

Time or Repetition:

- Beginner: Hold for 10 seconds.
- Intermediate: Hold for 20 seconds.
- Advanced: Hold for 30 seconds.

Cool Down: Slowly walk feet down the wall and rest in Child's Pose.

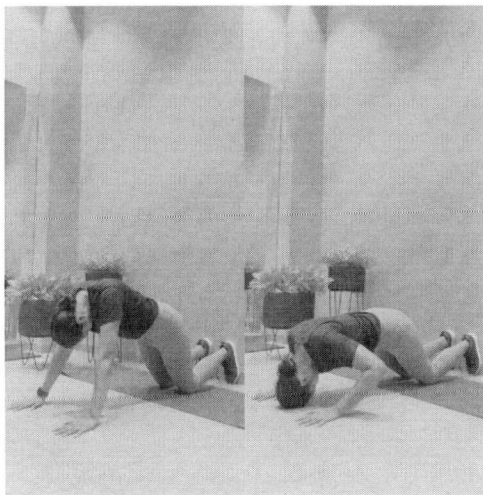

58. Wall Supported Pike Press

Scan for Video!

🎯 **Objective:** Increase shoulder and upper body strength, and improve flexibility in the hamstrings.

◎ **Focus:** Shoulders, upper body, hamstrings.

⚓ **Position:** Start in a Downward Dog position with your feet against the wall.

🧘 **Exercise:** Drop your knees straight down and place it on the floor, and bend your elbows to lower your head towards the ground, then straighten your elbow.

🧍 **Breathing:** Inhale as you lower, exhale as you press up.

⏱ **Time or Repetition:**

- Beginner: 5 repetitions.
- Intermediate: 8 repetitions.
- Advanced: 10 repetitions.

🧘 **Cool Down:** Rest in Child's Pose, stretching your arms forward.

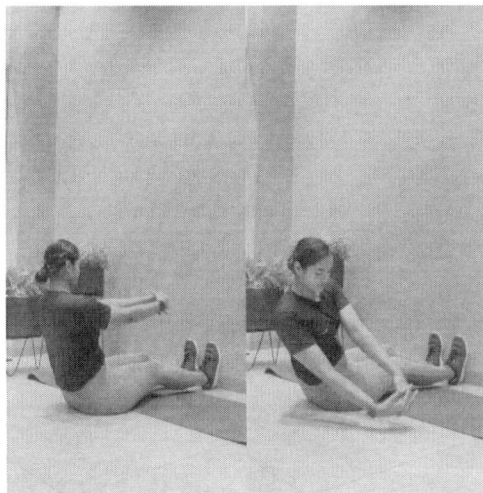

59. Wall Supported Boat Pose Twist

Scan for Video!

🎯 **Objective:** Strengthen the core, improve balance, and stimulate the digestive system.

◎ **Focus:** Core, balance, digestion.

⚓ **Position:** Sit perpendicular to the wall with your legs extended, lean back slightly, and lift your legs to form a V-shape.

🧘 **Exercise:** Twist your torso to touch the wall behind you with both hands, alternate sides.

🧍 **Breathing:** Inhale in the center, exhale as you twist.

⏱ **Time or Repetition:**

- Beginner: 5 twists each side.
- Intermediate: 8 twists each side.
- Advanced: 10 twists each side.

🧘 **Cool Down:** Hug your knees to your chest and gently rock side to side.

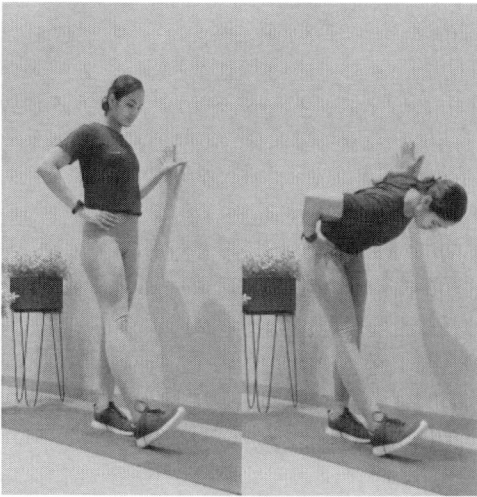

60. Wall Supported Pike Stretch

Scan for Video!

🎯 **Objective:** Increase flexibility in the hamstrings and lower back, improve circulation.

◎ **Focus:** Hamstrings, lower back.

⚓ **Position:** Stand facing the wall, feet hip-width apart, and lean forward to place your hands on the wall, keeping your legs straight.

💪 **Exercise:** Push your chest towards the floor to deepen the stretch in your hamstrings and back.

🧘 **Breathing:** Inhale as you lengthen the spine, exhale as you deepen the stretch.

⏱ **Time or Repetition:**

- Beginner: Hold for 20 seconds.

- Intermediate: Hold for 30 seconds.

- Advanced: Hold for 40 seconds.

🧘 **Cool Down:** Slowly roll up to standing, stretching upwards.

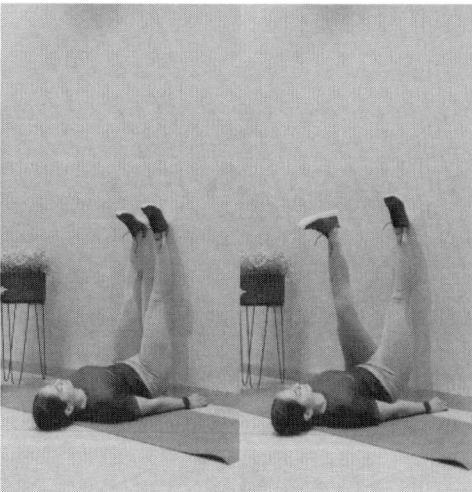

61. Wall Supported Leg Lifts

Scan for Video!

🎯 **Objective:** Strengthen the lower abdominals and improve hip flexor flexibility.

◎ **Focus:** Lower abdominals, hip flexors.

⚓ **Position:** Lie on your back with your legs against the wall, buttocks close to the wall.

💪 **Exercise:** Keep one leg on the wall while lowering the other leg towards the ground, then switch.

🧘 **Breathing:** Inhale as you lower the leg, exhale as you lift.

⏱ **Time or Repetition:**

- Beginner: 10 repetitions each leg.

- Intermediate: 15 repetitions each leg.

- Advanced: 20 repetitions each leg.

🧘 **Cool Down:** Rest both legs against the wall, deep breathing.

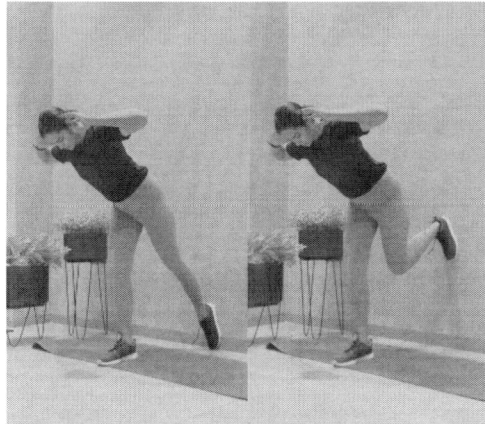

3.3 – For Advanced

62. Wall Supported Hamstring Curl

Scan for Video!

🎯 **Objective:** Strengthen the hamstrings and glutes, increase balance, and improve knee joint stability.

◎ **Focus:** Hamstrings, glutes, knee stability.

⚓ **Position:** Stand facing away from the wall, a short distance away, and lean forward after placing your hands behind your ear.

💪 **Exercise:** Bend one knee against the wall to bring your heel towards the ceiling, and perform a hamstring curl against the wall's resistance, then switch legs.

🧘 **Breathing:** Inhale as you bend the knee, exhale as you return to the starting position.

⏱ **Time or Repetition:**

- Beginner: 10 repetitions each leg.
- Intermediate: 15 repetitions each leg.
- Advanced: 20 repetitions each leg.

🧘 **Cool Down:** Gently stretch each leg by pulling the heel towards the glutes, standing upright.

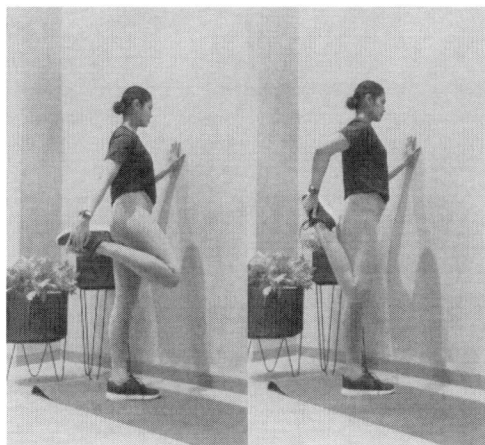

63. Wall Supported Quad Stretch

Scan for Video!

🎯 **Objective:** Enhance flexibility in the quadriceps and improve balance.

◎ **Focus:** Quadriceps, balance.

⚓ **Position:** Stand facing away from the wall, a short distance away. Bend one leg, bringing your heel towards your glutes, and grab your ankle with one hand.

💪 **Exercise:** Use the wall for balance as you gently pull your heel closer to your body to deepen the stretch in the quadriceps of the bent leg.

🧘 **Breathing:** Inhale as you prepare, exhale as you deepen the stretch.

⏱ **Time or Repetition:**

- Beginner: Hold for 20 seconds each leg.
- Intermediate: Hold for 30 seconds each leg.
- Advanced: Hold for 40 seconds each leg.

🧘 **Cool Down:** Gently release the leg, switch sides, and then relax both legs.

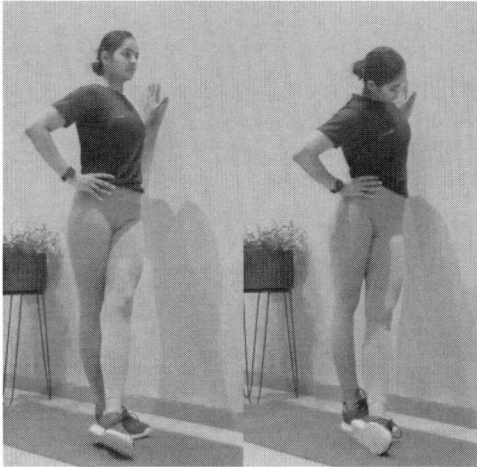

64. Wall Supported Hip Abductor Stretch

Scan for Video!

🎯 **Objective:** Increase flexibility in the hip abductors and improve hip mobility.

◎ **Focus:** Hip abductors, mobility.

⚓ **Position:** Stand sideways next to the wall, with the side of your body touching the wall. Cross the leg closest to the wall over the other leg.

💪 **Exercise:** Lean your hip towards the wall until you feel a stretch on the outer side of your hip.

🧘 **Breathing:** Inhale as you lean in, exhale as you hold the stretch.

⏱ **Time or Repetition:**

- Beginner: Hold for 20 seconds each side.
- Intermediate: Hold for 30 seconds each side.
- Advanced: Hold for 40 seconds each side.

🧘 **Cool Down:** Return to standing position, switch sides, and gently shake out the legs.

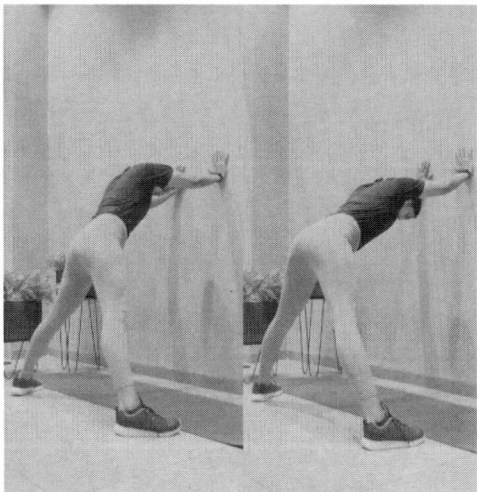

65. Wall Supported Hip Adductor Stretch

Scan for Video!

🎯 **Objective:** Improve flexibility in the inner thighs and enhance groin mobility.

◎ **Focus:** Hip adductors, inner thighs.

⚓ **Position:** Stand facing the wall, legs wide apart.

💪 **Exercise:** Lean forward towards the wall, allowing your legs to stretch apart until you feel a stretch in the inner thighs.

🧘 **Breathing:** Breathe deeply, focusing on relaxing the inner thigh muscles.

⏱ **Time or Repetition:**

- Beginner: Hold for 20 seconds.
- Intermediate: Hold for 30 seconds.
- Advanced: Hold for 40 seconds.

🧘 **Cool Down:** Slowly straighten up and bring legs together.

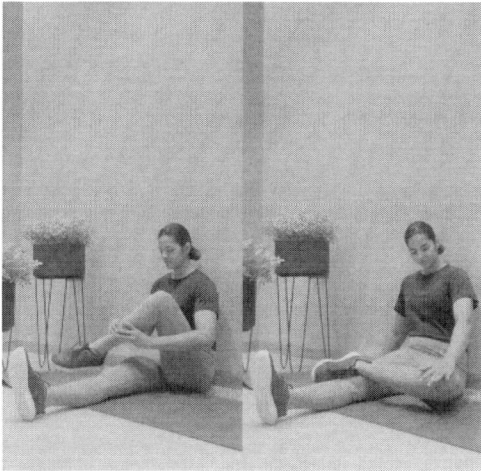

66. Wall-Supported Hip Internal Rotation Stretch

Scan for Video!

- ◎ **Objective:** Target the internal rotators of the hip for improved rotation mobility.
- ◎ **Focus:** Hip internal rotators, mobility.
- ⚓ **Position:** Sit with your back against the wall, legs extended in front of you. Bend one knee, placing the foot on the outside of the opposite knee.
- 👣 **Exercise:** Gently press the bent knee towards the floor, increasing the stretch as you maintain your back straight against the wall.

🧍 **Breathing:** Inhale as you prepare, exhale as you press the knee down.

⏱ **Time or Repetition:**

- Beginner: Hold for 20 seconds each side.
- Intermediate: Hold for 30 seconds each side.
- Advanced: Hold for 40 seconds each side.

🧘 **Cool Down:** Release the stretch gently, switch sides, and then extend both legs to relax.

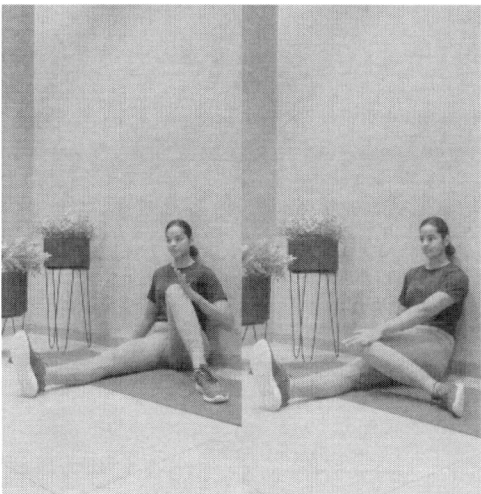

67. Wall-Supported Hip External Rotation Stretch

Scan for Video!

- ◎ **Objective:** Stretch the external rotators of the hips to enhance flexibility and reduce tightness.
- ◎ **Focus:** Hip external rotators, flexibility.
- ⚓ **Position:** Sit with your back against the wall, one leg bent at knee level away from the opposite leg.
- 👣 **Exercise:** Gently press the knees down towards the opposite knee to deepen the stretch, while keeping your spine straight against the wall and avoiding your buttocks coming off the floor.

🧍 **Breathing:** Inhale deeply, and exhale as you gently press the knees down.

⏱ **Time or Repetition:**

- Beginner: Hold for 20 seconds.
- Intermediate: Hold for 30 seconds.
- Advanced: Hold for 40 seconds.

🧘 **Cool Down:** Uncross the legs and gently shake them out in front of you.

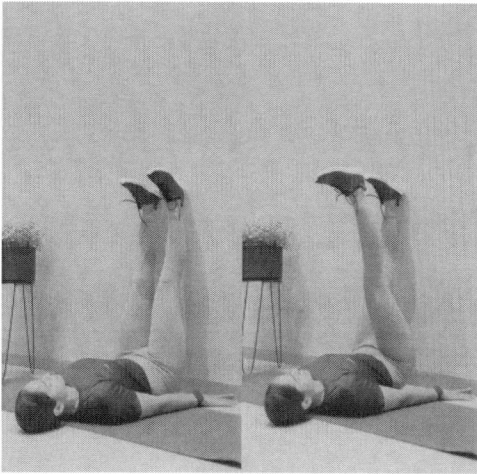

68. Wall Supported Leg Circles

Scan for Video!

🎯 **Objective:** Improve hip mobility and leg flexibility; strengthen hip flexors and leg muscles.

◎ **Focus:** Hips, leg muscles.

⚓ **Position:** Lie on your back with one leg raised against the wall and the other leg flat on the ground.

🤾 **Exercise:** Make circles in the air with the raised leg, keeping the movement controlled and the hip on the floor.

🧘 **Breathing:** Inhale to start the circle, exhale to complete it.

⏱ **Time or Repetition:**

- Beginner: 5 circles each direction, each leg.
- Intermediate: 8 circles each direction, each leg.
- Advanced: 10 circles each direction, each leg.

🧘 **Cool Down:** Lower the leg back to the starting position, switch legs, and then rest both legs on the ground.

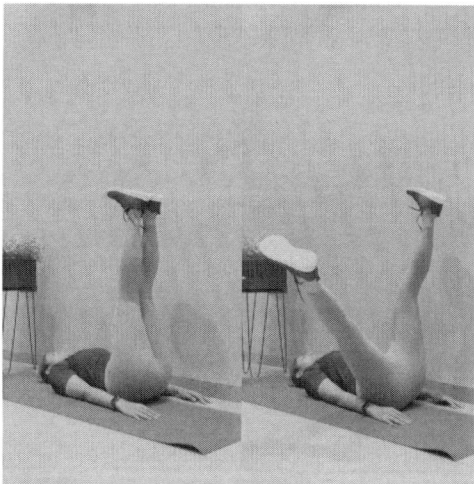

69. Wall Supported Leg Raise with Abduction

Scan for Video!

🎯 **Objective:** Strengthen the lower abdominals and improve lateral leg movement.

◎ **Focus:** Lower abdominals, outer thighs.

⚓ **Position:** Lie on your back parallel to the wall, with one side of your body closer to it. Lift both legs straight up towards the ceiling.

🤾 **Exercise:** Raise one leg upwards, then move it away from your body to the side (abduction) while keeping the other leg stationary.

🧘 **Breathing:** Inhale as you lift, exhale as you move the leg to the side.

⏱ **Time or Repetition:**

- Beginner: 5 repetitions each leg.
- Intermediate: 8 repetitions each leg.
- Advanced: 10 repetitions each leg.

🧘 **Cool Down:** Gently hug knees to chest and rock side to side.

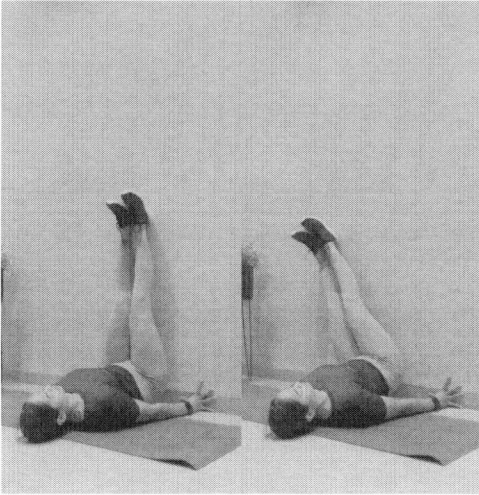

70. Wall Supported Leg Raise with Rotation

Scan for Video!

- 🎯 **Objective:** Increase core stability, enhance hip mobility, and strengthen the obliques.

- ◎ **Focus:** Core, hips, obliques.

- ⚓ **Position:** Lie on your back with your legs raised against the wall, feet together.

- 💪 **Exercise:** Keeping legs straight, rotate them side to side in a windshield wiper motion.

- 🧘 **Breathing:** Inhale in the center, exhale as you rotate to each side.

⏱ **Time or Repetition:**

- Beginner: 5 rotations each side.

- Intermediate: 8 rotations each side.

- Advanced: 10 rotations each side.

🧘 **Cool Down:** Rest legs up the wall, deep breathing to relax.

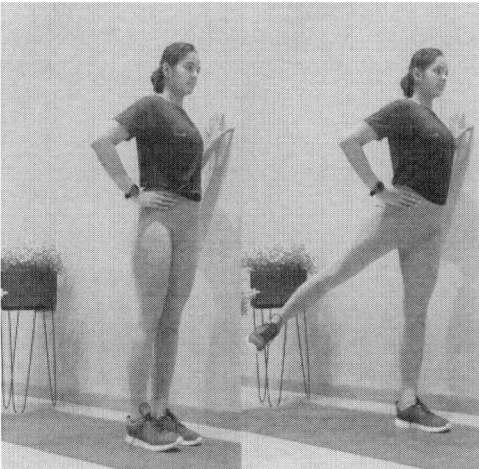

71. Wall Supported Leg Extension with Rotation

Scan for Video!

- 🎯 **Objective:** Enhance flexibility and strength in the legs, improve hip rotation.

- ◎ **Focus:** Legs, hips, core.

- ⚓ **Position:** Stand facing the wall, hands on the wall for balance.

- 💪 **Exercise:** Lift one leg straight back, then rotate the leg outward from the hip, and return to the center before lowering.

🧘 **Breathing:** Inhale as you lift and rotate, exhale as you return to the starting position.

⏱ **Time or Repetition:**

- Beginner: 5 repetitions each leg.

- Intermediate: 8 repetitions each leg.

- Advanced: 10 repetitions each leg.

🧘 **Cool Down:** Gently shake out each leg, then stretch both legs.

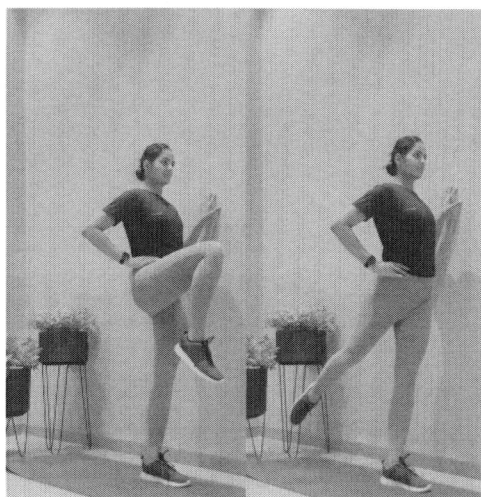

72. Wall Supported Leg Swing with Knee Flexion

Scan for Video!

🎯 **Objective:** Improve dynamic flexibility in the hamstrings, enhance knee and hip mobility.

◎ **Focus:** Hamstrings, knees, hips.

⚓ **Position:** Stand side-on to the wall, using it for support.

🧘 **Exercise:** Swing one leg forward with the knee bent, then extend the leg back in a controlled manner.

🧍 **Breathing:** Inhale as you swing forward, exhale as you swing back.

⏱ **Time or Repetition:**

- Beginner: 10 swings each leg.

- Intermediate: 15 swings each leg.

- Advanced: 20 swings each leg.

🧘 **Cool Down:** Stand still for a moment, then stretch the hamstrings and quads.

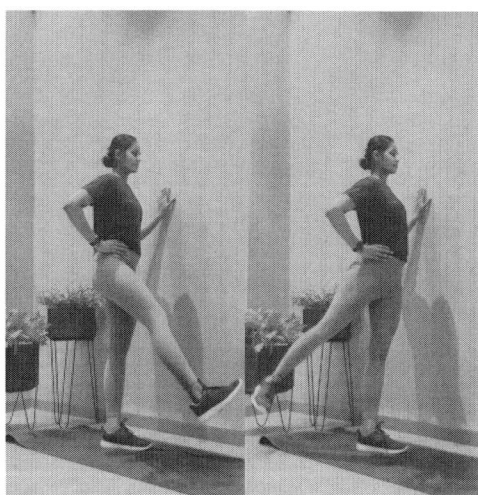

73. Wall Supported Leg Swing with Knee Extension

Scan for Video!

🎯 **Objective:** Increase leg flexibility, particularly in the hamstrings, and promote hip mobility.

◎ **Focus:** Hamstrings, hips.

⚓ **Position:** Face the wall, hands on the wall for support.

🧘 **Exercise:** Swing one straight leg forward and back in a pendulum motion, keeping the leg extended.

🧍 **Breathing:** Inhale as you swing forward, exhale as you swing back.

⏱ **Time or Repetition:**

- Beginner: 10 swings each leg.

- Intermediate: 15 swings each leg.

- Advanced: 20 swings each leg.

🧘 **Cool Down:** Gently stretch the legs by leaning forward, hands on the wall.

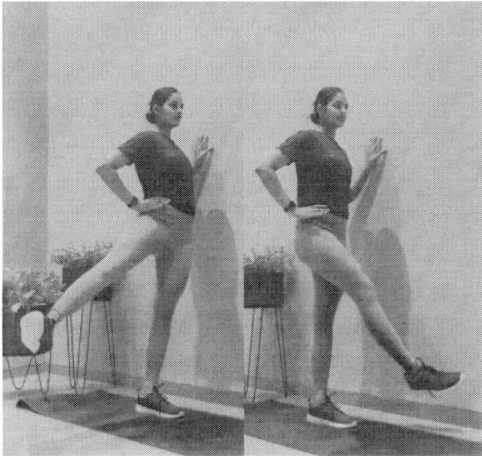

74. Wall Supported Leg Swing with Abduction

Scan for Video!

◎ **Objective:** Strengthen the outer thighs and hips, improve lateral mobility.

◎ **Focus:** Outer thighs, hips.

⚓ **Position:** Stand side-on to the wall, using it for balance.

☇ **Exercise:** Lift one leg out to the side, then swing it across your body in a controlled motion.

☇ **Breathing:** Inhale as you lift, exhale as you cross.

⏱ **Time or Repetition:**

- Beginner: 10 swings each leg.
- Intermediate: 15 swings each leg.
- Advanced: 20 swings each leg.

⟋ **Cool Down:** Stand still for a moment, then perform a gentle stretch for the outer thighs.

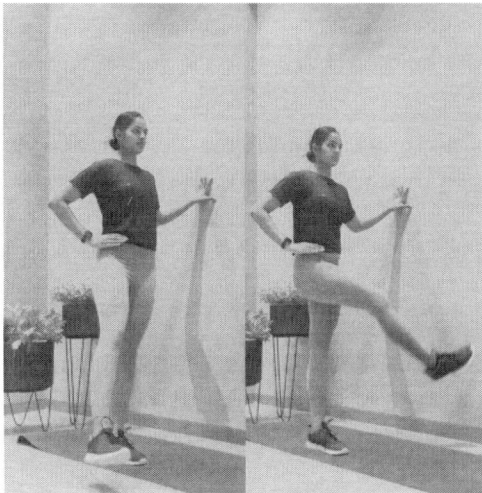

75. Wall Supported Leg Swing with Adduction

Scan for Video!

◎ **Objective:** Enhance inner thigh flexibility and strength, promote hip mobility.

◎ **Focus:** Inner thighs, hips.

⚓ **Position:** Stand away from the wall, holding onto it for support.

☇ **Exercise:** Swing one leg in front of the other, crossing your body, then swing it out to the side.

☇ **Breathing:** Inhale as you swing out, exhale as you swing across.

⏱ **Time or Repetition:**

- Beginner: 10 swings each leg.
- Intermediate: 15 swings each leg.
- Advanced: 20 swings each leg.

⟋ **Cool Down:** Relax the legs, gently stretch the inner thighs.

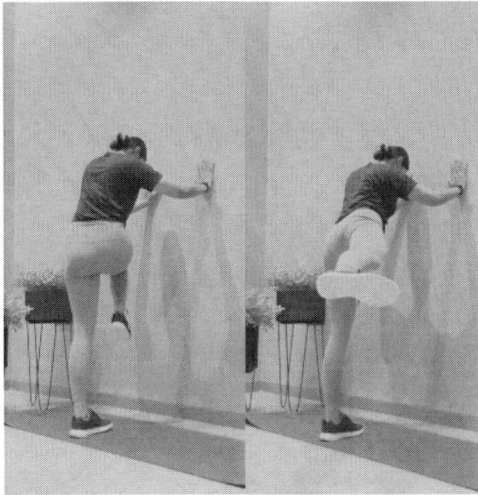

76. Wall Supported Leg Swing with Internal Rotation

Scan for Video!

🎯 **Objective:** Improve hip internal rotation mobility and flexibility in the legs.

◎ **Focus:** Hips, leg muscles.

⚓ **Position:** Stand facing the wall, lightly holding onto it for balance.

💪 **Exercise:** Lift one leg, knee bent, and rotate the hip inward, then swing the leg outward, keeping the rotation.

🧘 **Breathing:** Inhale as you rotate inward, exhale as you swing outward.

⏱ **Time or Repetition:**

- Beginner: 10 repetitions each leg.

- Intermediate: 15 repetitions each leg.

- Advanced: 20 repetitions each leg.

🧘 **Cool Down:** Gently shake out the legs, then stretch the hip rotators.

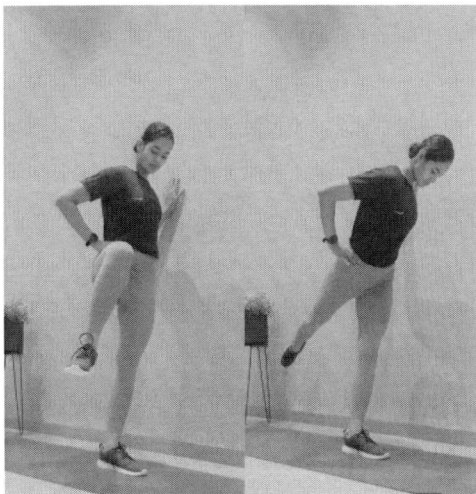

77. Wall Supported Leg Swing with External Rotation

Scan for Video!

🎯 **Objective:** Increase hip external rotation mobility, enhance flexibility across the hip joint.

◎ **Focus:** Hips, flexibility.

⚓ **Position:** Stand with your side to the wall, using it for balance.

💪 **Exercise:** Lift one leg, knee bent, and rotate the hip outward, then swing the leg inward, maintaining the rotation.

🧘 **Breathing:** Inhale as you rotate outward, exhale as you swing inward.

⏱ **Time or Repetition:**

- Beginner: 10 repetitions each leg.

- Intermediate: 15 repetitions each leg.

- Advanced: 20 repetitions each leg.

🧘 **Cool Down:** Stand still, then perform stretches focusing on hip mobility.

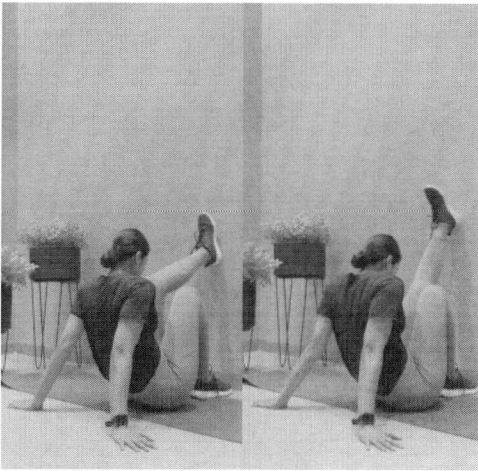

78. Wall Assisted Standing Split

Scan for Video!

⊙ **Objective:** Promote flexibility in the hamstrings and hips, improve balance.

⊙ **Focus:** Hamstrings, hips, balance.

⚓ **Position:** Face away from the wall, hands on the ground for support, one foot placed against the wall.

🤸 **Exercise:** Gently push your foot up the wall to deepen the standing split, aiming to increase flexibility over time.

🧘 **Breathing:** Inhale to prepare, exhale as you deepen the split.

⏱ **Time or Repetition:**

- Beginner: Hold for 20 seconds each leg.

- Intermediate: Hold for 30 seconds each leg.

- Advanced: Hold for 40 seconds each leg.

🧘 **Cool Down:** Carefully lower the leg, switch sides, then gently stretch both legs.

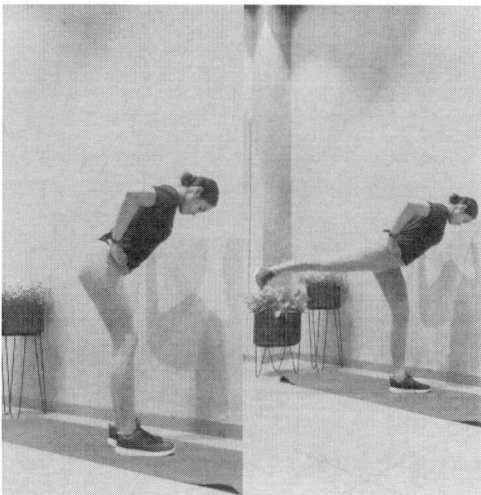

79. Wall Supported Side Kick Series

Scan for Video!

⊙ **Objective:** Strengthen the legs, glutes, and core; improve leg control and precision.

⊙ **Focus:** Legs, glutes, core.

⚓ **Position:** Stand side-on to the wall, using it for support.

🤸 **Exercise:** Perform a series of side kicks, focusing on control and precision. Include front kicks, side kicks, and back kicks in a controlled manner.

🧘 **Breathing:** Inhale to lift the leg, exhale as you perform the kick.

⏱ **Time or Repetition:**

- Beginner: 5 kicks each direction, each leg.

- Intermediate: 8 kicks each direction, each leg.

- Advanced: 10 kicks each direction, each leg.

🧘 **Cool Down:** Gently stretch the legs and hips, focusing on areas worked during the series.

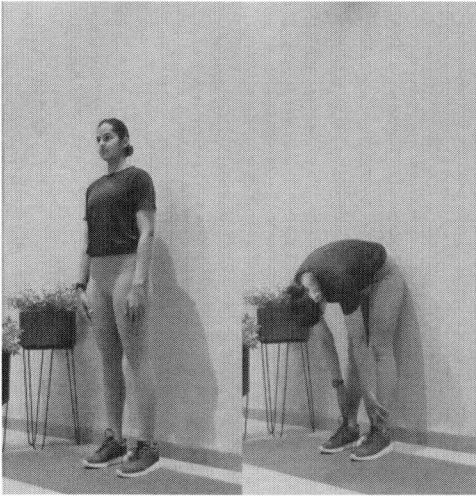

80. Wall Assisted Forward Fold

Scan for Video!

🎯 **Objective:** Increase flexibility in the hamstrings and lower back, and promote relaxation.

◎ **Focus:** Hamstrings, lower back.

⚓ **Position:** Stand a few inches away from the wall, feet hip-width apart.

💪 **Exercise:** Fold forward from the hips, reaching your hands down and sliding downwards to your feet. Allow your head to relax towards the floor, with the wall supporting your backside.

🧘 **Breathing:** Inhale as you fold, exhale as you deepen into the fold.

⏱ **Time or Repetition:**

- Beginner: Hold for 20 seconds.

- Intermediate: Hold for 30 seconds.

- Advanced: Hold for 40 seconds.

🧘 **Cool Down:** Slowly roll up to standing, taking deep breaths to relax.

81. Wall Climbing Stretch

Scan for Video!

🎯 **Objective:** Enhance overall flexibility and mimic climbing motion for improved upper body and core strength.

◎ **Focus:** Upper body, core, flexibility.

⚓ **Position:** Stand facing the wall, place your hands on the wall above your head.

💪 **Exercise:** "Climb" the wall with your hands, reaching up as high as possible, then walking them back down.

🧘 **Breathing:** Inhale as you reach up, exhale as you bring your hands down.

⏱ **Time or Repetition:**

- Beginner: 3 sets of 5 repetitions.

- Intermediate: 3 sets of 8 repetitions.

- Advanced: 3 sets of 10 repetitions.

🧘 **Cool Down:** Roll the shoulders and stretch the arms.

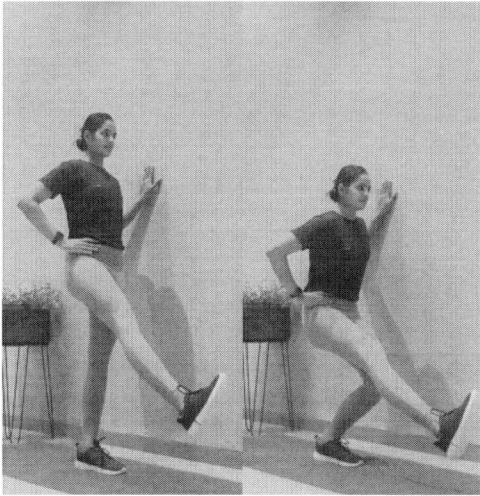

82. Wall Assisted Pistol Squat

Scan for Video!

🎯 **Objective:** Build strength and balance in the lower body, particularly focusing on one leg at a time.

◎ **Focus:** Quads, glutes, balance.

⚓ **Position:** Stand facing away from the wall, with one hand touching the wall for balance.

💪 **Exercise:** Lift one leg in front of you, and perform a squat on the standing leg, going as low as possible.

🧘 **Breathing:** Inhale on the way down, exhale on the way up.

⏱ **Time or Repetition:**

- Beginner: 5 repetitions each leg.

- Intermediate: 8 repetitions each leg.

- Advanced: 10 repetitions each leg.

🧘 **Cool Down:** Stretch both legs, focusing on the quads and hamstrings.

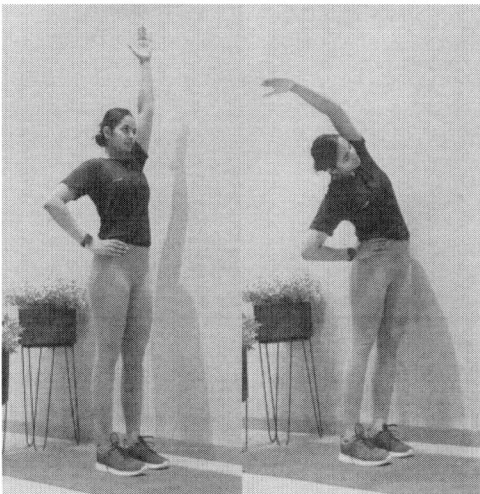

83. Wall Supported Side Stretch

Scan for Video!

🎯 **Objective:** Improve lateral flexibility in the torso, stretching the side muscles and enhancing mobility.

◎ **Focus:** Side torso, obliques.

⚓ **Position:** Stand with your side to the wall, feet together, reach the arm closest to the wall over your head.

💪 **Exercise:** Lean towards the wall, stretching the side of your body away from the wall.

🧘 **Breathing:** Inhale to reach up, exhale as you stretch towards the wall.

⏱ **Time or Repetition:**

- Beginner: Hold for 20 seconds each side.

- Intermediate: Hold for 30 seconds each side.

- Advanced: Hold for 40 seconds each side.

🧘 **Cool Down:** Return to standing and gently twist the torso to release tension.

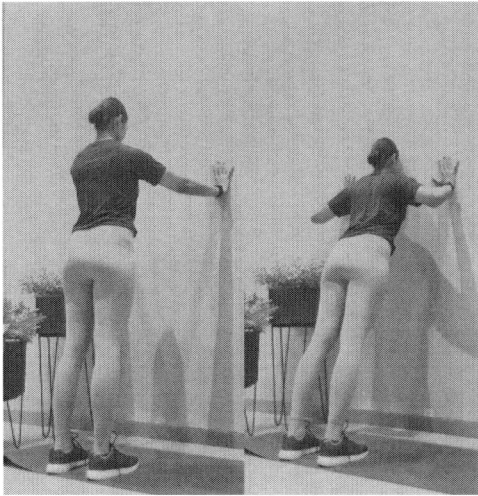

84. Wall Push-Away

Scan for Video!

🎯 **Objective:** Strengthen the chest, shoulders, and arms with dynamic pushing movement.

◎ **Focus:** Chest, shoulders, triceps.

⚓ **Position:** Stand facing the wall, place both hands on it slightly wider than shoulder-width apart.

💪 **Exercise:** Lean into the wall, bending your elbows, then push yourself back to the starting position with force.

🧍 **Breathing:** Inhale as you lean in, exhale as you push away.

🕐 **Time or Repetition:**

- Beginner: 10 repetitions.

- Intermediate: 15 repetitions.

- Advanced: 20 repetitions.

🧘 **Cool Down:** Shoulder rolls and arm stretches.

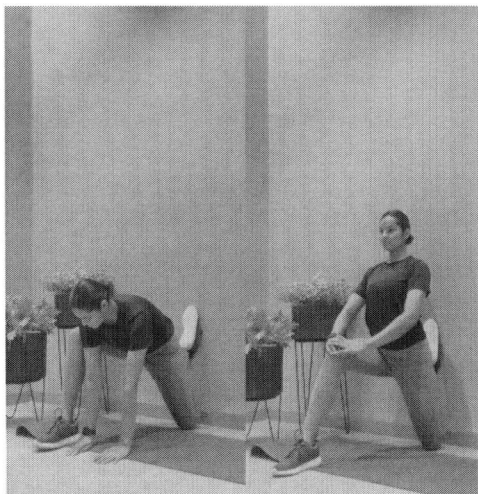

85. Wall Lunge Stretch

Scan for Video!

🎯 **Objective:** Increase flexibility in the hip flexors and thighs, improve balance.

◎ **Focus:** Hip flexors, thighs.

⚓ **Position:** Stand facing away from the wall, one foot placed back against the wall.

💪 **Exercise:** Bend the front knee into a lunge position, keeping the back leg straight and the heel pressing against the wall.

🧍 **Breathing:** Inhale as you lower into the lunge, exhale as you hold.

🕐 **Time or Repetition:**

- Beginner: Hold for 20 seconds each side.

- Intermediate: Hold for 30 seconds each side.

- Advanced: Hold for 40 seconds each side.

🧘 **Cool Down:** Gently release the lunge and switch sides.

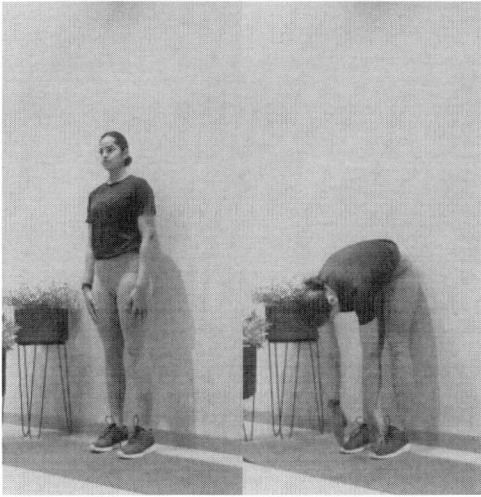

86. Wall Assisted Toe Touch

Scan for Video!

🎯 **Objective:** Enhance flexibility in the hamstrings and lower back, and promote relaxation.

◎ **Focus:** Hamstrings, lower back.

⚓ **Position:** Stand a foot away from the wall, legs straight.

💪 **Exercise:** Bend forward from the hips, trying to touch your toes or the floor directly without support, with the wall touching your backside at the end range.

🧍 **Breathing:** Inhale as you start to bend, exhale as you reach down.

⏱ **Time or Repetition:**

- Beginner: Hold for 20 seconds.

- Intermediate: Hold for 30 seconds.

- Advanced: Hold for 40 seconds.

🧘 **Cool Down:** Slowly roll up to standing, stretching upwards.

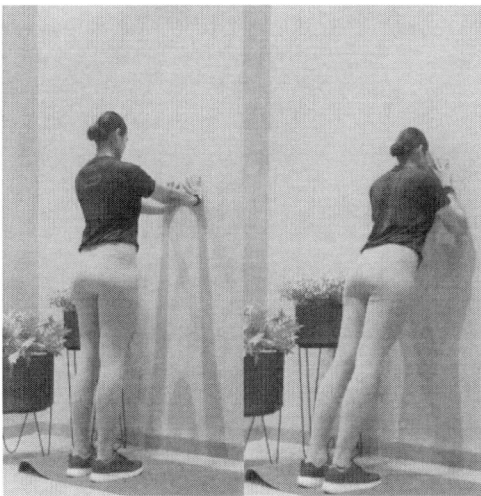

87. Wall Diamond Push-Up

Scan for Video!

🎯 **Objective:** Target the triceps and inner chest with a challenging push-up variation.

◎ **Focus:** Triceps, inner chest.

⚓ **Position:** Face the wall, hands on the wall forming a diamond shape (index fingers and thumbs touching).

💪 **Exercise:** Bend your elbows to lower your chest towards the wall, then push back to the starting position.

🧍 **Breathing:** Inhale as you lower, exhale as you push back.

⏱ **Time or Repetition:**

- Beginner: 8 repetitions.

- Intermediate: 12 repetitions.

- Advanced: 15 repetitions.

🧘 **Cool Down:** Stretch the chest and arms.

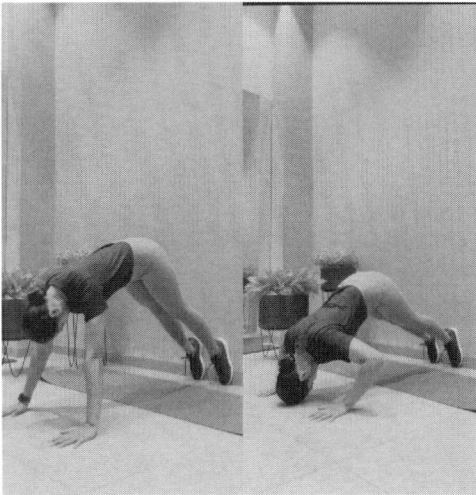

88. Wall Inverted Shoulder Press

Scan for Video!

🎯 **Objective:** Strengthen the shoulders and upper back with an inverted position.

◎ **Focus:** Shoulders, upper back.

⚓ **Position:** Start in a pike position with feet on the wall, hands on the ground.

💪 **Exercise:** Lower your head towards the ground by bending the elbows, then press back up.

🧘 **Breathing:** Inhale as you lower, exhale as you press up.

⏱ **Time or Repetition:**

- Beginner: 5 repetitions.

- Intermediate: 8 repetitions.

- Advanced: 10 repetitions.

🧘 **Cool Down:** Gently come down and rest in Child's Pose.

89. Wall Assisted Corkscrew

Scan for Video!

🎯 **Objective:** Improve core strength and oblique engagement with rotational movements.

◎ **Focus:** Core, obliques.

⚓ **Position:** Lie on your back with legs raised against the wall, arms out for balance.

💪 **Exercise:** Rotate your hips to move your legs in a circular motion, mimicking a corkscrew.

🧘 **Breathing:** Coordinate breathing with the movement, inhaling as legs go up, exhaling as they rotate.

⏱ **Time or Repetition:**

- Beginner: 5 circles each direction.

- Intermediate: 8 circles each direction.

- Advanced: 10 circles each direction.

🧘 **Cool Down:** Hug knees to chest, gently rock side to side.

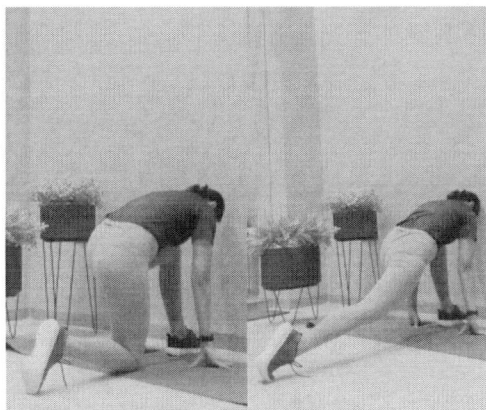

90. Wall Supported Standing Split

Scan for Video!

- **Objective:** Increase flexibility in the hamstrings and hips, improve balance.

- **Focus:** Hamstrings, hips, balance.

- **Position:** Stand with your back to the wall, hands on the floor, one leg lifted and foot placed against the wall.

- **Exercise:** Push into the wall with the lifted foot to increase the split depth.

Breathing: Inhale as you lift the leg, exhale as you deepen the split.

Time or Repetition:

- Beginner: Hold for 20 seconds each leg.

- Intermediate: Hold for 30 seconds each leg.

- Advanced: Hold for 40 seconds each leg.

Cool Down: Gently lower the leg, switch sides, and relax.

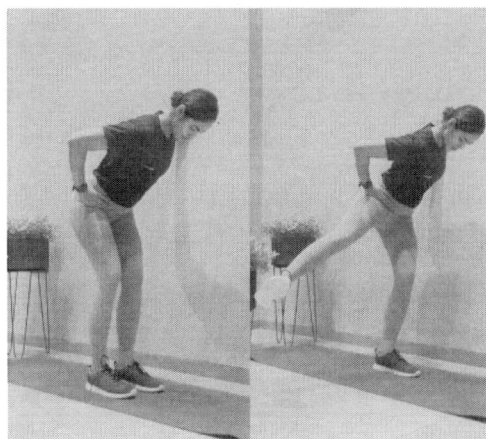

91. Wall Supported Hip Hinge with Leg Lift

Scan for Video!

- **Objective:** Improve lower back strength, enhance leg and core stability, and mimic the lateral leg movement benefits similar to the Wall Supported Side Kick Series.

- **Focus:** Lower back, legs, core stability.

- **Position:** Stand perpendicular to the wall with one hand for support. Feet should be hip-width apart, with the side closer to the wall slightly behind you for balance.

Exercise: Bend at the hips to lean forward into a hinge position, keeping your back straight. Lift the leg furthest from the wall to the side in a controlled manner, then lower it back down.

Breathing: Inhale as you hinge and prepare, exhale as you lift the leg.

Time or Repetition:

- Beginner: 5 lifts each leg.

- Intermediate: 8 lifts each leg.

- Advanced: 10 lifts each leg.

Cool Down: Stand upright and perform gentle leg and hip stretches, focusing on the muscles worked during the exercise.

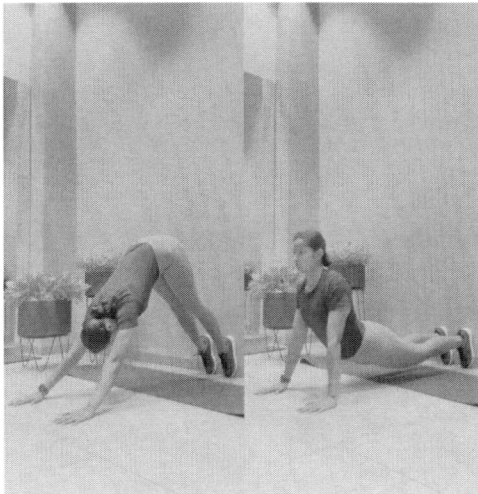

92. Wall-Assisted Swing Push-up

Scan for Video!

🎯 **Objective:** Strengthen shoulders and upper back, increase flexibility in hamstrings.

◎ **Focus:** Shoulders, upper back, hamstrings.

⚓ **Position:** Start in a high plank with feet against the wall, hands on the ground shoulder-width apart.

💪 **Exercise:** Push hips upwards, forming an inverted V shape with your body, keeping feet on the wall. Drop hips down to the floor gently, coming to a cobra position before restarting the sequence.

🧘 **Breathing:** Inhale as you lift your hips, exhale as you lower.

⏱ **Time or Repetition:**

- **Beginner**: 3 repetitions.
- **Intermediate**: 5 repetitions.
- **Advanced**: 8 repetitions.

🧘 **Cool Down:** Return to a high plank position, then gently step down to a kneeling position to rest.

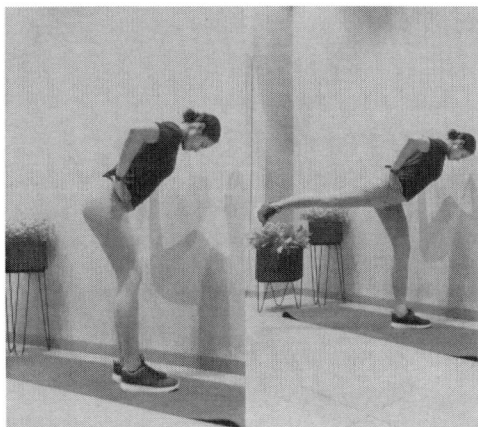

93. Wall-Supported Single-Leg Deadlift

Scan for Video!

🎯 **Objective:** Improve balance and strengthen the lower back, glutes, and hamstrings.

◎ **Focus:** Lower back, glutes, hamstrings.

⚓ **Position:** Stand facing away from the wall, lightly touching it with one hand for balance. Stand on one leg.

💪 **Exercise:** Hinge at the hips to lower your torso forward while lifting the opposite leg straight behind you, touching the wall for balance.

🧘 **Breathing:** Inhale as you lower, exhale as you return to standing.

⏱ **Time or Repetition:**

- **Beginner**: 5 repetitions per leg.
- **Intermediate**: 8 repetitions per leg.
- **Advanced**: 12 repetitions per leg.

🧘 **Cool Down:** Stand upright and shake out the legs gently.

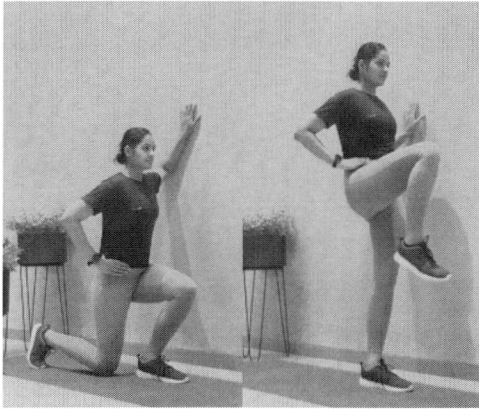

94. Wall-Assisted Reverse Lunge with Knee Drive

Scan for Video!

🎯 **Objective:** Enhance lower body strength and stability, improve knee lift height.

◎ **Focus:** Quadriceps, glutes, core.

⚓ **Position:** Stand facing away from the wall, a few feet in front.

💪 **Exercise:** Step back with one foot into a reverse lunge, lightly touching the wall for balance. Explosively drive the same knee upwards as you return to standing.

🧎 **Breathing:** Inhale during the lunge, exhale as you drive the knee up.

⏱ **Time or Repetition:**

- **Beginner**: 5 repetitions per leg.
- **Intermediate**: 8 repetitions per leg.
- **Advanced**: 12 repetitions per leg.

🧘 **Cool Down:** Gentle leg stretches.

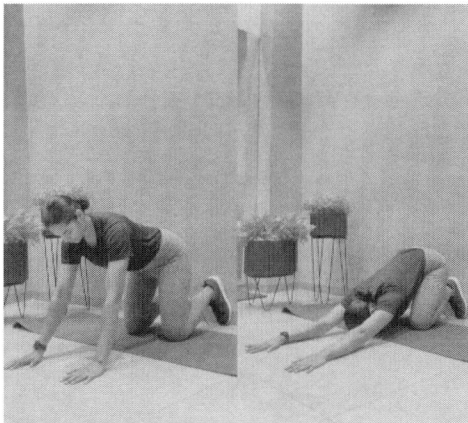

95. Wall-Supported Puppy Pose

Scan for Video!

🎯 **Objective:** Increase shoulder flexibility, improve shoulder joint health.

◎ **Focus:** Shoulders, core.

⚓ **Position:** Start in an all 4's position with ankles flat on the wall close to the ground.

💪 **Exercise:** Drop your chest to the floor as low as possible while simultaneously sliding hands away from you, keeping lower body position as it is.

🧎 **Breathing:** Maintain steady breathing throughout.

⏱ **Time or Repetition:**

- **Beginner**: 3 repetitions.
- **Intermediate**: 5 repetitions.
- **Advanced**: 8 repetitions.

🧘 **Cool Down:** Return to the floor and rest in child's pose.

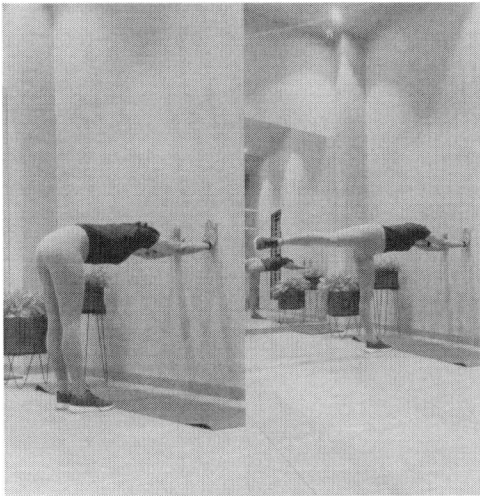

96. Wall-Supported Warrior III

Scan for Video!

🎯 **Objective:** Improve balance and strengthen the posterior chain.

◎ **Focus:** Glutes, hamstrings, lower back.

⚓ **Position:** Stand facing away from the wall, placing hands on the wall at hip height for balance.

💪 **Exercise:** Lean forward into a Warrior III pose, extending one leg straight back and arms forward, keeping hands on the wall.

🧎 **Breathing:** Inhale as you lean forward, exhale as you return to standing.

⏱ **Time or Repetition:**

- **Beginner:** Hold for 5 seconds per leg.
- **Intermediate:** Hold for 10 seconds per leg.
- **Advanced:** Hold for 15 seconds per leg.

🧎 **Cool Down:** Stand upright and shake out the legs gently.

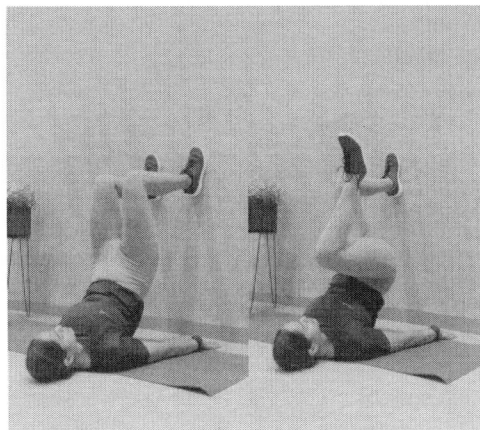

97. Wall-Assisted Glute Bridge Single-Leg March

Scan for Video!

🎯 **Objective:** Strengthen the glutes and hamstrings, improve balance.

◎ **Focus:** Glutes, hamstrings, core.

⚓ **Position:** Lie on your back with feet flat against the wall, knees bent. Lift into a glute bridge position.

💪 **Exercise:** March by alternating lifting each foot off the wall while keeping your hips elevated and stable.

🧎 **Breathing:** Inhale on the lift, exhale as you lower the foot back to the wall.

⏱ **Time or Repetition:**

- **Beginner:** 5 marches with each leg, maintaining the bridge.
- **Intermediate:** 10 marches with each leg, hold the bridge.
- **Advanced:** 15 marches with each leg, add a pause at the top of each march.

🧎 **Cool Down:** Lower hips to the floor and stretch the hamstrings.

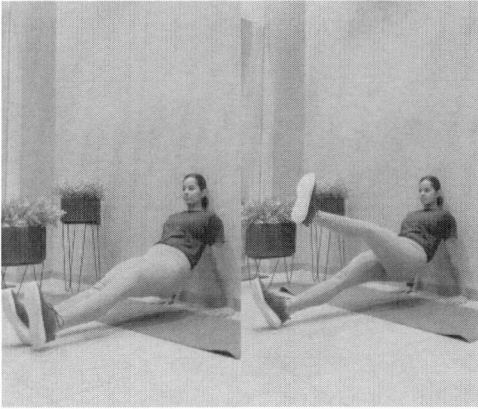

98. Wall-Assisted Reverse Plank Leg Lift

Scan for Video!

🎯 **Objective:** Increase core strength and stability, enhance shoulder endurance.

◎ **Focus:** Core, shoulders, glutes.

⚓ **Position:** Sit facing away from the wall, hands on the ground behind you, feet against the wall.

💪 **Exercise:** Lift into a reverse plank, then alternately lift each leg.

🧘 **Breathing:** Inhale to lift the leg, exhale to lower.

⏱ **Time or Repetition:**

- **Beginner**: Alternate leg lifts for 5 reps each leg.
- **Intermediate**: Alternate leg lifts for 10 reps each leg with a higher lift.
- **Advanced**: Alternate leg lifts for 15 reps each leg, hold each lift for 3 seconds.

🧘 **Cool Down:** Sit down gently and stretch your shoulders and hamstrings.

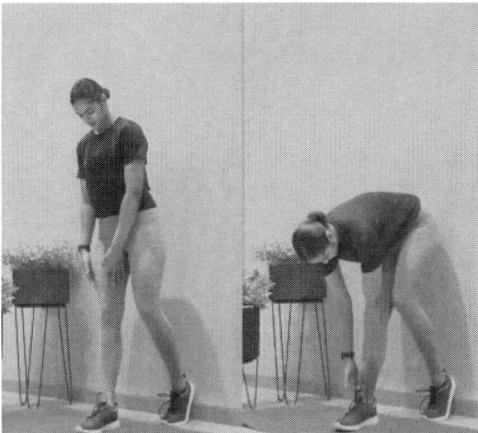

99. Wall-Assisted Single Leg Hamstring Stretch

Scan for Video!

🎯 **Objective:** Strengthen hamstrings and improve posterior chain flexibility.

◎ **Focus:** Hamstrings, calves, glutes.

⚓ **Position:** Stand close to the wall facing away from it. Bend one knee and support it with the wall.

💪 **Exercise:** Slowly lean forward towards the straightened leg using your hands to "crawl"/"slide" towards the end, keeping your knees straight. Go as low as possible before you come up to the starting position. Repeat on the other leg.

🧘 **Breathing:** Inhale on the way down, exhale to push back up.

⏱ **Time or Repetition:**

- **Beginner**: 3-5 reps with a moderate lean.
- **Intermediate**: 5-8 reps with a deeper lean.
- **Advanced**: 8-10 reps, going as low as possible.

🧘 **Cool Down:** Stretch your hamstrings and calves.

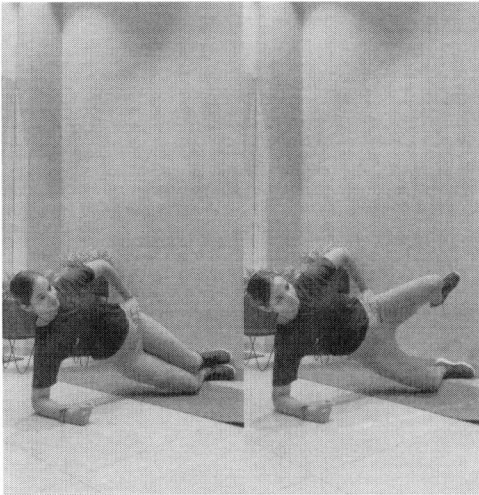

100. Wall-Supported Modified Side Plank with Leg Lift

Scan for Video!

🎯 **Objective:** Improve lateral core stability and strengthen the abductors.

◎ **Focus:** Core, obliques, glutes.

⚓ **Position:** Start in a modified side plank position with your feet against the wall, knees bent, close to the ground.

💪 **Exercise:** Lift the top leg in the same knee angle, while maintaining the side plank position.

🧘 **Breathing:** Inhale to lift the leg slightly, exhale to lower.

⏱ **Time or Repetition:**

- **Beginner**: Hold plank for 10 seconds, 5 leg lifts.

- **Intermediate**: Hold plank for 20 seconds, 10 leg lifts.

- **Advanced**: Hold plank for 30 seconds, 15 leg lifts with a pause at the top.

🧘 **Cool Down:** Transition to a seated position and gently stretch the sides of your body.

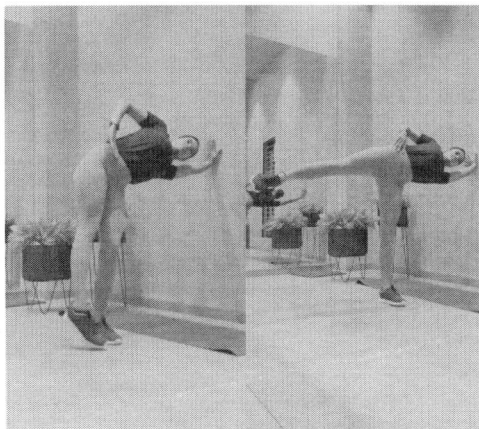

101. Wall-Supported Half Moon Pose

Scan for Video!

🎯 **Objective:** Enhance balance and lateral flexibility, strengthen the legs and core.

◎ **Focus:** Core, glutes, obliques.

⚓ **Position:** Start in a standing position, leaning into the wall with one hand fully extended, other hand on your hip, and feet together.

💪 **Exercise:** Lift your foot away from wall towards the ceiling, while tilting your body sideways, aiming to form a straight line from the lifted foot to the top hand.

🧘 **Breathing:** Inhale as you extend into the pose, exhale to deepen the stretch.

⏱ **Time or Repetition:**

- **Beginner**: Hold the pose for 10 seconds on each side.

- **Intermediate**: Hold for 20 seconds on each side, aim for a greater stretch.

- **Advanced**: Hold for 30 seconds on each side, focus on lifting the leg higher and reaching further with the top hand.

🧘 **Cool Down:** Return to standing and do gentle side stretches.

3.4 – Exercises divided by Benefits

Whether you're looking to improve your core strength, boost your flexibility, or achieve better posture, there's a Wall Pilates exercise perfect for you!

Exercises for Warm-Up

Wall Roll Down (1)

Scan for Video!

Wall Pelvic Tilt (13)

Scan for Video!

Scan for Video!

Wall Shoulder Rolls (11)

Scan for Video!

Wall Arm Slides (9)

Wall Neck Extensions (12)

Scan for Video!

Exercises for Strength and Stability

Wall Supported Hundred (2)

Scan for Video!

Wall Push-Up (17)

Scan for Video!

Scan for Video!

Wall Reverse Plank (6)

Scan for Video!

Wall Supported Side Plank (25)

Wall Supported Bridge (7)

Scan for Video!

Scan for Video!

Wall Supported Plank with Leg Raise (37)

Scan for Video!

Wall Plank (15)

Scan for Video!

Wall Mountain Climbers (40)

Wall Jump Squats (51)

Scan for Video!

Scan for Video!

Wall Burpees (55)

Wall Push Away (84)

Scan for Video!

Wall Diamond Push-Up (87)

Wall Inverted Shoulder Press (88)

Scan for Video!

Wall-Assisted Glute Bridge Single-Leg March (97)

Scan for Video!

Scan for Video!

Wall-Assisted Reverse Plank Leg Lift (98)

Wall-Assisted Single Leg Hamstring Stretch (99)

Scan for Video!

Exercises for Flexibility and Mobility

Wall Supported Bicycle (3)

Scan for Video!

Scan for Video!

Wall Single Leg Slide (4)

Wall Standing Leg Circles (5)

Scan for Video!

Scan for Video!

Wall Supported Ankle Stretches (22)

Wall Supported Flexibility Routine (26)

Scan for Video!

Scan for Video!

Wall Supported Fish Pose (28)

Wall Supported Child's Pose (29)

Scan for Video!

Scan for Video!

Wall Supported Spinal Twist (30)

Scan for Video!

Wall Supported Shoulder
Stand (31)

Scan for Video!

Wall Pigeon Pose (34)

Scan for Video!

Wall Supported Bycicle (35)

Scan for Video!

Wall Supported Downward
Facing Dog (36)

Scan for Video!

Wall Supported Bridge
Lift (56)

Scan for Video!

Wall Supported Boat Pose
Twist (59)

Scan for Video!

Wall Supported Pike
Stretch (60)

Scan for Video!

Wall Supported Hip
Abductor Stretch (64)

Scan for Video!

Wall Supported Hip
Adductor Stretch (65)

Scan for Video!

Wall Supported Hip Internal
Rotation Stretch (66)

Scan for Video!

Wall Supported Hip External
Rotation Stretch (67)

Scan for Video!

Wall Supported Leg
Circles (68)

Scan for Video!

Wall Supported Leg Raise
with Abduction (69)

Scan for Video!

Wall Supported Leg Raise
with Rotation (70)

Scan for Video!

Wall Supported Leg
Extension
with Rotation (71)

Scan for Video!

Wall Supported Side
Stretch (83)

Scan for Video!

Wall Lunge Stretch (85)

Scan for Video!

Wall-Supported Half Moon
Pose (101)

Exercises for Core and Balance

Wall Supported Core Workout (38)

Scan for Video!

Wall Supported Hamstring Curl (62)

Scan for Video!

Scan for Video!

Wall Supported Balance Challenge (39)

Scan for Video!

Wall Supported Quad Stretch (63)

Wall Supported Headstand (57)

Scan for Video!

Wall-Supported Puppy Pose (95)

Scan for Video!

Scan for Video!

Wall Supported Pike Press (58)

Scan for Video!

Wall-Supported Modified Side Plank with Leg Lift (100)

Wall Supported Leg Lifts (61)

Scan for Video!

Exercises for Relaxation and Stress Relief

Wall Supported Relaxation (27)

Scan for Video!

Wall Supported Spinal Twist (30)

Scan for Video!

Scan for Video!

Wall Supported Child's Pose (29)

Scan for Video!

Wall Supported Shoulder Stand (31)

Cardiovascular and Endurance

Wall Scissor Kicks (41)

Scan for Video!

Wall High Knees (53)

Scan for Video!

Scan for Video!

Wall Flutter Kicks (42)

Scan for Video!

Wall Tuck Jumps (54)

Exercises for Dynamic Flexibility

Wall Downward Dog (14)

Scan for Video!

Wall Standing Leg Extension (47)

Scan for Video!

Scan for Video!

Wall Hamstring Stretch (16)

Scan for Video!

Wall Pike (48)

Wall Sit with Leg Raise (18)

Scan for Video!

Wall Mermaid Pose (49)

Scan for Video!

Scan for Video!

Wall Deep Sit (8)

Scan for Video!

Wall Pike Slides (50)

Wall Supported Warrior II (44)

Scan for Video!

Wall Oblique Twists (52)

Scan for Video!

Scan for Video!

Wall Supported Squat Slide (45)

Scan for Video!

Wall Marching (43)

Wall-Assisted Swing Push-Up (92)

Scan for Video!

Wall Roll Over (46)

Scan for Video!

Scan for Video!

Wall-Assisted Reverse Lunge with Knee Drive (94)

Exercises for Posture and Alignment

Wall Chest Opener (10)

Scan for Video!

Scan for Video!

Wall Tree Pose (19)

Wall Butterfly Stretch (20)

Scan for Video!

Wall Palms Slide (21)

Scan for Video!

Wall Assisted Knee Lifts (23)

Scan for Video!

Wall Assisted Calf Raises (24)

Scan for Video!

Wall Triangle Pose (32)

Scan for Video!

Wall Warrior Pose (33)

Scan for Video!

Wall Supported Leg Swing with Knee Flexion (72)

Scan for Video!

Wall Supported Leg Swing with Knee Extension (73)

Wall Supported Leg Swing with Abduction (74)

Scan for Video!

Scan for Video!

Wall Supported Leg Swing with Adduction (75)

Wall Supported Leg Swing with Internal Rotation (76)

Scan for Video!

Scan for Video!

Wall Supported Leg Swing with External Rotation (77)

Wall Assisted Standing Split (78)

Scan for Video!

Scan for Video!

Wall Supported Side Kick Series (79)

Wall Assisted Forward Fold (80)

Scan for Video!

Scan for Video!

Wall Climbing Stretch (81)

Wall Assisted Pistol Squat (82)

Scan for Video!

Scan for Video!

Wall Assisted Toe Touch (86)

Scan for Video!

Wall Assisted Corkscrew (89)

Wall Supported Split
Progression (90)

Scan for Video!

Wall Supported Hip Hinge
with Leg Lift (91)

Scan for Video!

Wall-Supported Single-Leg
Deadlift (93)

Scan for Video!

Wall-Supported Warrior III (96)

Scan for Video!

ARE YOU ENJOYING THE BOOK?

Leave your HONEST REVIEW

to GREATLY support my path as an author.

Thank YOU so much!

Elevate your Wall Pilates journey with these **specially designed bonuses**. Access them directly with ease:

Bonus 1: 7-Day No Stress Meal Plan.

Carefully crafted to complement your Wall Pilates routine, these meals are designed to nourish your body and soothe your soul.

Scan for PDF!

SCAN this QR code

Bonus 2: 8-Week Challenge.

This Challenge is designed to give you a boost, not only in your physical health but also in your mental and emotional well-being.

Scan for PDF!

SCAN this QR code

Bonus 3: 10 Mindfulness Exercises.

These exercises are tailored to seniors, aiming to improve concentration, enhance emotional equilibrium, and promote a sense of present-moment awareness.

Scan for PDF!

SCAN this QR code

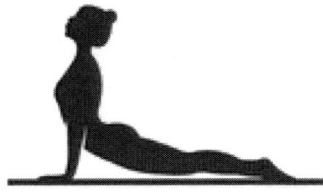

Chapter 4:
4 Routines for Everyday Practice

"A few well-designed movements, properly performed in a balanced sequence, are worth hours of doing sloppy calisthenics or forced contortion."

Joseph Pilates

4.1 - 5 Minutes Wake-Up Routine

We all want to wake up and face each day with a body that is alert, alert, and prepared to take on any task. This morning routine provides exactly that: a sequence of somewhat challenging but highly effective exercises designed to shift your body from a state of rest to one of preparation. Your daily workout should not be replaced by this practice; rather, it should be used to prime your muscles, improve circulation, and correct your posture. By doing these exercises, you'll discover the best method to awaken your body, make sure you're ready for the day both mentally and physically.

For Beginners

1. Wall Roll Down (1)
   - 1 minute

Scan for Video!

2. Wall Arm Slides (9)
   - 1 minute

Scan for Video!

3. Wall Shoulder Rolls (11)
   - 1 minute

Scan for Video!

4. Wall Pelvic Tilt (13)
   - 1 minute

Scan for Video!

5. Wall Hamstring Stretch (16)
   - 1 minute

Scan for Video!

For Intermediate

1. Wall Supported Hundred (2) - 1 minute

2. Wall Downward Dog (14) - 1 minute

3. Wall Supported Bicycle (3) - 1 minute

4. Wall Standing Leg Circles (5) - 1 minute

5. Wall Chest Opener (10) - 1 minute

For Advanced

1. Wall Supported Plank with Leg Raise (37) - 1 minute

2. Wall Supported Warrior II (44) - 1 minute

3. Wall Supported Hamstring Curl (62) - 1 minute

4. Wall Pike (48) - 1 minute

5. Wall Climbing Stretch (81) - 1 minute

4.2 - 5 Minutes Warm-Up Routine

Any successful exercise program must begin with a proper warm-up, but this is especially true with Wall Pilates. By improving blood flow to the muscles and boosting flexibility, it modifies your body's readiness for the impending physical activity and lowers your chance of injury. In addition to helping, you focus and synchronize your breathing with your actions, a well-planned warm-up regimen also mentally readies you for exercise. You can guarantee a safer, more effective, and more satisfying Wall Pilates practice by allocating a few minutes to warm up.

For Beginners

1. Wall Roll Down (1)
- 1 minute

Scan for Video!

2. Wall Arm Slides (9)
- 1 minute

3. Wall Shoulder Rolls (11)
- 1 minute

4. Wall Pelvic Tilt (13)
- 1 minute

Scan for Video!

5. Wall Hamstring Stretch (16) - 1 minute

For Intermediate

1. Wall Roll Down (1) - 1 minute

2. Wall Arm Slides (9)
- 1 minute

3. Wall Neck Extensions (12)
- 1 minute

4. Wall Downward Dog (14)
- 1 minute

5. Wall Butterfly Stretch (20) - 1 minute

For Advanced

1. Wall Roll Down (1) - 1 minute

2. Wall Arm Slides (9)
- 1 minute

3. Wall Chest Opener (10)
- 1 minute

4. Wall Supported Leg Circles (68) - 1 minute

5. Wall Climbing Stretch (81) - 1 minute

4.3 – 5 minutes Sweet Dreams Routine

Achieving a deep, restorative sleep requires calming your body and mind before going to bed. It can be difficult to properly wind down in the daily chaos. But the secret to achieving a restful night's sleep may lie in a focused muscle relaxation regimen created especially with Wall Pilates principles. This workout regimen is designed to help you go asleep more easily by gradually calming your body, easing your mind, and releasing any physical or mental tension.

For Beginners

1. Wall Supported Child's Pose (29) - 1 minute

2. Wall Supported Spinal Twist (30) - 1 minute

3. Wall Pelvic Tilt (13) - 1 minute

4. Wall Supported Relaxation (27) - 2 minutes

For Intermediate

1. Wall Supported Fish Pose (28) - 1 minute

2. Wall Butterfly Stretch (20) - 1 minute

3. Wall Supported Child's Pose (29) - 1 minute

4. Wall Supported Leg Lifts (61) - 1 minute

5. Wall Supported Relaxation (27) - 1 minute

For Advanced

1. Wall Supported Child's Pose (29) - 1 minute

2. Wall Supported Spinal Twist (30) - 1 minute

3. Wall Supported Bridge Lift (56) - 1 minute

4. Wall Supported Hip External Rotation Stretch (67) - 1 minute

5. Wall Supported Relaxation (27) - 1 minute

4.4 - 15 Minutes Daily Workout Routine for 7 Days

Welcome to a fun 7-day Wall Pilates experience designed specifically for you and your everyday routine. I have just the thing for you whether you're ready to push yourself to the limit, are trying to add more depth to your current Pilates practice, or are just getting started in the realm of fitness. Envision a sequence of movements, carefully selected to correspond with your current fitness level and intended to provide you with enjoyment, difficulty, and a feeling of achievement.

For a week, how about setting aside only 15 minutes each day for yourself? In the time it might take to sip a cup of tea, you can learn what your body is capable of, feel stronger and more flexible, and declutter your mind—all while exercising.

For Beginners

Day 1: Building Core Strength

Warm-Up (5 minutes):

1. Wall Arm Slides (9) - 1 minute

2. Wall Shoulder Rolls (11) - 1 minute

3. Wall Neck Extensions (12) - 1 minute

4. Wall Hamstring Stretch (16) - 2 minutes (1 minute each leg)

Flexibility and Mobility (5 minutes):

1. Wall Pelvic Tilt (13) - 2 minutes

2. Wall Supported Spinal Twist (30) - 2 minutes

3. Wall Butterfly Stretch (20) - 1 minute

Relaxation and Stress Relief (5 minutes):

1. Wall Supported Relaxation (27) - 2 minutes

2. Wall Supported Child's Pose (29) - 2 minutes

3. Wall Supported Fish Pose (28) - 1 minute

Day 2: Enhancing Flexibility

Warm-Up (5 minutes):

1. Wall Shoulder Rolls (11) - 2 minutes

Scan for Video!

2. Wall Neck Extensions (12) - 1 minute

Scan for Video!

3. Wall Pelvic Tilt (13) - 2 minutes

Scan for Video!

Flexibility and Mobility (5 minutes):

1. Wall Downward Dog (14) - 2 minutes

Scan for Video!

2. Wall Butterfly Stretch (20) - 2 minutes

Scan for Video!

3. Wall Supported Ankle Stretches (22) - 1 minute

Scan for Video!

Relaxation and Stress Relief (5 minutes):

1. Wall Supported Child's Pose (29) - 2 minutes

Scan for Video!

2. Wall Supported Fish Pose (28) - 2 minutes

Scan for Video!

3. Wall Supported Relaxation (27) - 1 minute

Scan for Video!

Day 3: Lower Body Strength

Warm-Up (5 minutes):

1. Wall Arm Slides (9)
   - 2 minutes

2. Wall Pelvic Tilt (13) -
   1 minute

3. Wall Hamstring Stretch
   (16) - 2 minutes

Strength and Stability (5 minutes):

1. Wall Sit with Leg Raise (18)
   - 2 minutes (1 minute each leg)

2. Wall Supported Bridge (7)
   - 2 minutes

3. Wall Assisted Calf
   Raises (24) - 1 minute

Relaxation and Stress Relief (5 minutes):

1. Wall Supported Child's
   Pose (29) - 2 minutes

2. Wall Supported Fish Pose
   (28) - 2 minutes

3. Wall Supported
   Relaxation (27) - 1 minute

Day 4: Upper Body and Core Focus

Warm-Up (5 minutes):

1. Wall Neck Extensions (12) - 1 minute

Scan for Video!

2. Wall Shoulder Rolls (11) - 2 minutes

3. Wall Arm Slides (9) - 2 minutes

Scan for Video!

Strength and Stability (5 minutes):

1. Wall Plank (15) - 2 minutes

Scan for Video!

2. Wall Push-Up (17) - 2 minutes

3. Wall Supported Side Plank (25) - 1 minute (30 seconds each side)

Scan for Video!

Relaxation and Stress Relief (5 minutes):

1. Wall Supported Child's Pose (29) - 2 minutes

Scan for Video!

2. Wall Supported Relaxation (27) - 2 minutes

3. Wall Supported Fish Pose (28) - 1 minute

Scan for Video!

Day 5: Posture and Alignment

Warm-Up (5 minutes):

1. Wall Arm Slides (9) - 2 minutes

Scan for Video!

3. Wall Neck Extensions (12) - 2 minutes

Scan for Video!

Scan for Video!

2. Wall Shoulder Rolls (11) - 1 minute

Flexibility and Mobility (5 minutes):

1. Wall Tree Pose (19) - 2 minutes (1 minute each side)

Scan for Video!

3. Wall Palms Slide (21) - 1 minute

Scan for Video!

Scan for Video!

2. Wall Chest Opener (10) - 2 minutes

Relaxation and Stress Relief (5 minutes):

1. Wall Supported Fish Pose (28) - 2 minutes

Scan for Video!

3. Wall Supported Relaxation (27) - 1 minute

Scan for Video!

Scan for Video!

2. Wall Supported Child's Pose (29) - 2 minutes

Day 6: Full Body Engagement

Warm-Up (5 minutes):

1. Wall Hamstring Stretch (16) - 2 minutes (1 minute each leg)

2. Wall Arm Slides (9) - 1 minute

3. Wall Shoulder Rolls (11) - 2 minutes

Strength and Stability (5 minutes):

1. Wall Reverse Plank (6) - 2 minutes

2. Wall Push-Up (17) - 2 minutes

3. Wall Supported Hundred (2) - 1 minute

Relaxation and Stress Relief (5 minutes):

1. Wall Supported Child's Pose (29) - 2 minutes

2. Wall Supported Relaxation (27) - 2 minutes

3. Wall Supported Fish Pose (28) - 1 minute

Day 7: Balance and Coordination

Warm-Up (5 minutes):

1. Wall Shoulder Rolls (11) - 2 minutes

2. Wall Neck Extensions (12) - 1 minute

3. Wall Arm Slides (9) - 2 minutes

Core and Balance (5 minutes):

1. Wall Tree Pose (19) - 2 minutes (1 minute each side)

2. Wall Plank (15) - 2 minutes

3. Wall Supported Ankle Stretches (22) - 1 minute

Relaxation and Stress Relief (5 minutes):

1. Wall Supported Relaxation (27) - 2 minutes

2. Wall Supported Child's Pose (29) - 2 minutes

3. Wall Supported Fish Pose (28) - 1 minute

For Intermediate

Day 1: Core and Upper Body Strength

Warm-Up (5 minutes):

1. Wall Arm Slides (9) - 1 minute

2. Wall Chest Opener (10) - 2 minutes

3. Wall Neck Extensions (12) - 2 minutes

Strength and Stability (5 minutes):

1. Wall Supported Hundred (2) - 2 minutes

2. Wall Push-Up (17) - 2 minutes

3. Wall Supported Plank with Leg Raise (37) - 1 minute

Relaxation and Stress Relief (5 minutes):

1. Wall Supported Child's Pose (29) - 2 minutes

2. Wall Supported Relaxation (27) - 3 minutes

Day 2: Flexibility and Leg Strength

Warm-Up (5 minutes):

1. Wall Hamstring Stretch (16) - 2 minutes (1 minute each leg)

2. Wall Pelvic Tilt (13) - 2 minutes

3. Wall Shoulder Rolls (11) - 1 minute

Flexibility and Mobility (5 minutes):

1. Wall Pigeon Pose (34) - 2 minutes (1 minute each side)

Scan for Video!

Scan for Video!

2. Wall Supported Ankle Stretches (22) - 2 minutes

3. Wall Butterfly Stretch (20) - 1 minute

Scan for Video!

Relaxation and Stress Relief (5 minutes):

1. Wall Supported Fish Pose (28) - 2 minutes

Scan for Video!

Scan for Video!

2. Wall Supported Child's Pose (29) - 3 minutes

Day 3: Balance and Core Focus

Warm-Up (5 minutes):

1. Wall Arm Slides (9) - 1 minute

Scan for Video!

Scan for Video!

2. Wall Neck Extensions (12) - 2 minutes

3. Wall Shoulder Rolls (11) - 2 minutes

Scan for Video!

Core and Balance (5 minutes):

1. Wall Supported Balance Challenge (39) - 2 minutes

Scan for Video!

Scan for Video!

2. Wall Triangle Pose (32) - 2 minutes (1 minute each side)

3. Wall Warrior Pose (33) - 1 minute

Scan for Video!

Relaxation and Stress Relief (5 minutes):

1. Wall Supported Relaxation (27) - minutes

2. Wall Supported Child's Pose (29) - 3 minutes

Day 4: Cardio and Lower Body Strength

Warm-Up (5 minutes):

1. Wall Hamstring Stretch (16) - 2 minutes (1 minute each leg)

3. Wall Shoulder Rolls (11) - 2 minutes

2. Wall Pelvic Tilt (13) - 1 minute

Cardiovascular and Endurance (5 minutes):

1. Wall Mountain Climbers (40) - 2 minutes

3. Wall Tuck Jumps (54) - 1 minute

2. Wall High Knees (53) - 2 minutes

Relaxation and Stress Relief (5 minutes):

1. Wall Supported Child's Pose (29) - 2 minutes

2. Wall Supported Relaxation (27) - 3 minutes

Day 5: Dynamic Flexibility and Mobility

Warm-Up (5 minutes):

1. Wall Arm Slides (9) - 1 minute

3. Wall Shoulder Rolls (11) - 2 minutes

2. Wall Neck Extensions (12) - 2 minutes

Flexibility and Mobility (5 minutes):

1. Wall Downward Dog (14) - 2 minutes

3. Wall Supported Pike Stretch (60) - 1 minute

2. Wall Supported Downward Facing Dog (36) - 2 minutes

Relaxation and Stress Relief (5 minutes):

1. Wall Supported Fish Pose (28) - 2 minutes

2. Wall Supported Child's Pose (29) - 3 minutes

Day 6: Core Intensive

Warm-Up (5 minutes):

1. Wall Arm Slides (9) - 1 minute

3. Wall Neck Extensions (12) - 2 minutes

2. Wall Chest Opener (10) - 2 minutes

Strength and Stability (5 minutes):

1. Wall Supported Core Workout (38) - 2 minutes

Scan for Video!

3. Wall Supported Leg Lifts (61) - 1 minute

Scan for Video!

Scan for Video!

2. Wall Plank (15) - 2 minutes

Relaxation and Stress Relief (5 minutes):

1. Wall Supported Child's Pose (29) - 2 minutes

Scan for Video!

Scan for Video!

2. Wall Supported Relaxation (27) - 3 minutes

Day 7: Full Body Workout

Warm-Up (5 minutes):

1. Wall Shoulder Rolls (11) - 1 minute

Scan for Video!

3. Wall Pelvic Tilt (13) - 2 minutes

Scan for Video!

Scan for Video!

2. Wall Neck Extensions (12) - 2 minutes

Mixed Focus (5 minutes):

1. Wall Reverse Plank (6) - 2 minutes

Scan for Video!

3. Wall Mermaid Pose (49) - 1 minute

Scan for Video!

Scan for Video!

2. Wall Supported Bridge (7) - 2 minutes

Relaxation and Stress Relief (5 minutes):

1. Wall Supported Fish Pose (28) - 2 minutes

   Scan for Video!

   Scan for Video!

2. Wall Supported Child's Pose (29) - 3 minutes

For Advanced
Day 1: Advanced Core Challenge
Warm-Up (5 minutes):

1. Wall Arm Slides (9) - 1 minute

   Scan for Video!

3. Wall Pelvic Tilt (13) - 2 minutes

   Scan for Video!

   Scan for Video!

2. Wall Chest Opener (10) - 2 minutes

Core Intensity (5 minutes):

1. Wall Supported Core Workout (38) - 2 minutes

   Scan for Video!

3. Wall Supported Leg Lifts (61) - 1 minute

   Scan for Video!

   Scan for Video!

2. Wall Supported Pike Press (58) - 2 minutes

Flexibility Cool-Down (5 minutes):

1. Wall Supported Pike Stretch (60) - 2 minutes

   Scan for Video!

   Scan for Video!

2. Wall Supported Quad Stretch (63) - 3 minutes

Day 2: Leg Strength and Mobility

Warm-Up (5 minutes):

1. Wall Neck Extensions (12) - 1 minute

   Scan for Video!

3. Wall Supported Ankle Stretches (22) - 2 minutes

   Scan for Video!

   Scan for Video!

2. Wall Hamstring Stretch (16) - 2 minutes (1 minute each leg)

Strength and Stability (5 minutes):

1. Wall Assisted Pistol Squat (82) - 2 minutes (1 minute each leg)

   Scan for Video!

3. Wall Assisted Calf Raises (24) - 1 minute

   Scan for Video!

   Scan for Video!

2. Wall Supported Hamstring Curl (62) - 2 minutes

Mobility and Stretch (5 minutes):

1. Wall Supported Hip Abductor Stretch (64) - 2 minutes

   Scan for Video!

   Scan for Video!

2. Wall Supported Hip Adductor Stretch (65) - 3 minutes

Day 3: Balance and Flexibility Focus

Warm-Up (5 minutes):

1. Wall Shoulder Rolls (11) - 2 minutes

   Scan for Video!

3. Wall Downward Dog (14) - 2 minutes

   Scan for Video!

   Scan for Video!

2. Wall Pelvic Tilt (13) - 1 minute

Balance and Flexibility (5 minutes):

1. Wall Supported Balance Challenge (39) - 2 minutes

Scan for Video!

2. Wall Supported Split Progression (90) - 2 minutes

3. Wall Supported Side Stretch (83) - 1 minute

Scan for Video!

Relaxation (5 minutes):

1. Wall Supported Relaxation (27) - 5 minutes

Scan for Video!

Day 4: Upper Body Strength

Warm-Up (5 minutes):

1. Wall Arm Slides (9) - 1 minute

Scan for Video!

2. Wall Chest Opener (10) - 2 minutes

3. Wall Pelvic Tilt (13) - 2 minutes

Scan for Video!

Upper Body Power (5 minutes):

1. Wall Push-Up (17) - 2 minutes

Scan for Video!

2. Wall Diamond Push-Up (87) - 2 minutes

3. Wall Inverted Shoulder Press (88) - 1 minute

Scan for Video!

Stretch and Recovery (5 minutes):

1. Wall Supported Child's Pose (29) - 2 minutes

    Scan for Video!

2. Wall Supported Fish Pose (28) - 3 minutes

    Scan for Video!

Day 5: Dynamic Stretching and Strength

Warm-Up (5 minutes):

1. Wall Shoulder Rolls (11) - 1 minute

    Scan for Video!

3. Wall Neck Extensions (12) - 2 minutes

    Scan for Video!

2. Wall Pelvic Tilt (13) - 2 minutes

    Scan for Video!

Dynamic Movement (5 minutes):

1. Wall Supported Leg Swing with Knee Flexion (72) - 2 minutes

    Scan for Video!

3. Wall Supported Leg Swing with External Rotation (77) - 1 minute

    Scan for Video!

2. Wall Supported Leg Swing with Abduction (74) - 2 minutes

    Scan for Video!

Cool-Down (5 minutes):

1. Wall Supported Relaxation (27) - 2 minutes

    Scan for Video!

2. Wall Supported Spinal Twist (30) - 3 minutes

    Scan for Video!

Day 6: Comprehensive Body Workout

Warm-Up (5 minutes):

1. Wall Arm Slides (9) - 2 minutes

2. Wall Neck Extensions (12) - 1 minute

3. Wall Pelvic Tilt (13) - 2 minutes

Full Body Challenge (5 minutes):

1. Wall Burpees (55) - 2 minutes

2. Wall Supported Headstand (57) - 2 minutes

3. Wall Climbing Stretch (81) - 1 minute

Stretch and Relaxation (5 minutes):

1. Wall Supported Relaxation (27) - 2 minutes

2. Wall Supported Child's Pose (29) - 3 minutes

Day 7: Flexibility and Control

Warm-Up (5 minutes):

1. Wall Shoulder Rolls (11) - 2 minutes

2. Wall Hamstring Stretch (16) - 2 minutes (1 minute each leg)

3. Wall Pelvic Tilt (13) - 1 minute

Flexibility Focus (5 minutes):

1. Wall Supported Hip External Rotation Stretch (67) - 2 minutes

Scan for Video!

3. Wall Supported Leg Raise with Rotation (70) - 1 minute

Scan for Video!

Scan for Video!

2. Wall Supported Boat Pose Twist (59) - 2 minutes

Relaxation and Mindfulness (5 minutes):

1. Wall Supported Relaxation (27) - 2 minutes

Scan for Video!

Scan for Video!

2. Wall Supported Fish Pose (28) - 3 minutes

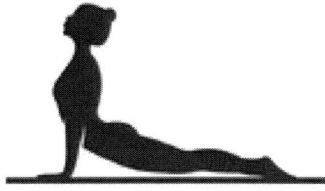

Chapter 5:
28-Day Challenge

"Change happens through movement, and movement heals."

Joseph Pilates

Are you ready to transform your body and mind in just one month?

This challenge is designed to help you build strength, flexibility, and balance while improving your posture and overall health.

Over the next 28 days, you will follow a daily workout routine that incorporates a variety of Wall Pilates exercises. These exercises are designed to target all major muscle groups and can be modified to fit your fitness level.

What you will need:

- A yoga mat

- A wall

- A water bottle

- Comfortable workout clothes

What you can expect:

- Each workout will take approximately 15 minutes to complete.

- You will work out 7 days a week, with no rest day.

- The workouts will gradually increase in intensity as you progress.

Benefits:

- Improved strength and flexibility

- Better posture and alignment

- Increased balance and coordination

- Reduced stress and anxiety

Here are some additional tips for success:

- Set realistic goals for yourself.

- Listen to your body and take breaks when needed.

- Stay hydrated and eat a healthy diet.

- Celebrate your progress along the way!

Are you ready to take the challenge?

Start your journey to a healthier and happier you by selecting from one of the following 3 categories based on your experience with wall Pilates, your physical fitness, and any physical limitations that may restrict your mobility.

5.1 – For Beginners

Scan for Video!

Week 1: Foundation and Flexibility

Weekly Goal: Introduce foundational poses to gently increase flexibility and encourage mindfulness.

Daily Routine (10 minutes):

Pause for 20-30 seconds before moving on to the next exercise

- **Warm-Up:**

  - **Wall Supported Relaxation (27)** - 3 minutes

- **Wall Roll Down (1)** - 5 repetitions

- **Wall Supported Spinal Twist (30)** - 3 repetitions each side

- **Wall Supported Flexibility Routine (26)** - Hold for 20 seconds

- **Wall Pelvic Tilt (13)** - 5 repetitions

- **Wall Hamstring Stretch (16)** - Hold for 20 seconds each side

- **Wall Butterfly Stretch (20)** - Hold for 20 seconds

- **Cool-Down:**

  - **Wall Supported Child's Pose (29)** - 3 minutes

Week 2: Building Strength

Weekly Goal: Start building core and lower body strength to improve posture and stability.

Daily Routine (10 minutes):

Pause for 20-30 seconds before moving on to the next exercise

- **Warm-Up:**
    - **Wall Arm Slides (9)** - 3 minutes
- **Wall Supported Bridge (7)** - Hold for 20 seconds, 5 repetitions
- **Wall Sit with Leg Raise (18)** - Hold each leg for 20 seconds, alternate legs
- **Wall Push-Up (17)** - 5 repetitions
- **Wall Plank (15)** - Hold for 20 seconds
- **Wall Supported Side Plank (25)** - Hold for 20 seconds each side
- **Wall Assisted Calf Raises (24)** - 10 repetitions
- **Cool-Down:**
    - **Wall Supported Relaxation (27)** - 3 minutes

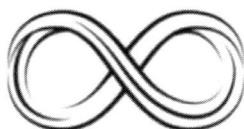

Week 3: Enhancing Balance and Coordination

Weekly Goal: Focus on exercises that enhance balance and coordination, key for everyday activities.

Daily Routine (10 minutes):

Pause for 20-30 seconds before moving on to the next exercise

- **Warm-Up:**
    - **Wall Neck Extensions (12)** - 3 minutes
- **Wall Tree Pose (19)** - Hold for 20 seconds each side
- **Wall Supported Balance Challenge (39)** - 5 repetitions
- **Wall Standing Leg Circles (5)** - 5 repetitions each leg
- **Wall Supported Bicycle (3)** - 10 repetitions each side
- **Wall Single Leg Slide (4)** - 5 repetitions each leg
- **Wall Palms Slide (21)** - Hold for 20 seconds
- **Cool-Down:**
    - **Wall Supported Fish Pose (28)** - 3 minutes

Week 4: Mindfulness and Relaxation

Weekly Goal: Emphasize mindfulness and relaxation techniques to enhance mental well-being alongside physical fitness.

Daily Routine (10 minutes):

Pause for 20-30 seconds before moving on to the next exercise

- **Warm-Up:**
  - **Wall Shoulder Rolls (11)** - 3 minutes
- **Wall Supported Child's Pose (29)** - Hold for 20 seconds
- **Wall Supported Spinal Twist (30)** - 3 repetitions each side
- **Wall Downward Dog (14)** - Hold for 20 seconds
- **Wall Chest Opener (10)** - Hold for 20 seconds
- **Wall Neck Extensions (12)** - 5 repetitions
- **Wall Supported Ankle Stretches (22)** - Hold for 20 seconds each side
- **Cool-Down:**
  - **Wall Supported Relaxation (27)** - 3 minutes

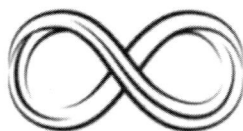

Scan for Video!

5.2 – For Intermediate

Week 1: Core Strengthening

Weekly Goal: Focus on strengthening the core muscles, which are vital for overall stability and strength.

Daily Routine (10 minutes):

Pause for 20-30 seconds before moving on to the next exercise

- **Warm-Up:**
  - **Wall Arm Slides (9)** - 3 minutes
- **Wall Supported Hundred (2)** - 5 repetitions
- **Wall Supported Plank with Leg Raise (37)** - 10 repetitions each side
- **Wall Mountain Climbers (40)** - 10 repetitions each side
- **Wall Supported Core Workout (38)** - Hold for 20 seconds
- **Wall Scissor Kicks (41)** - 10 repetitions
- **Wall Flutter Kicks (42)** - 10 repetitions
- **Cool-Down:**
  - **Wall Supported Relaxation (27)** - 3 minutes

Scan for Video!

Week 2: Flexibility and Mobility Enhancement

Weekly Goal: Improve flexibility and mobility with a focus on stretching and dynamic movements.

Scan for Video!

Daily Routine (10 minutes):

Pause for 20-30 seconds before moving on to the next exercise

- **Warm-Up:**
    - **Wall Neck Extensions (12)** - 3 minutes
- **Wall Pigeon Pose (34)** - Hold for 20 seconds each side
- **Wall Supported Downward Facing Dog (36)** - Hold for 20 seconds
- **Wall Supported Warrior II (44)** - Hold for 20 seconds each side
- **Wall Supported Boat Pose Twist (59)** - 10 repetitions
- **Wall Supported Pike Stretch (60)** - Hold for 20 seconds
- **Wall Butterfly Stretch (20)** - Hold for 20 seconds
- **Cool-Down:**
    - **Wall Supported Fish Pose (28)** - 3 minutes

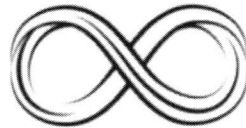

Week 3: Building Lower Body Strength

Weekly Goal: Enhance lower body strength through focused exercises on legs, glutes, and calves.

Scan for Video!

Daily Routine (10 minutes):

Pause for 20-30 seconds before moving on to the next exercise

- **Warm-Up:**
    - **Wall Pelvic Tilt (13)** - 3 minutes
- **Wall Supported Squat Slide (45)** - 10 repetitions
- **Wall Jump Squats (51)** - 10 repetitions
- **Wall Supported Leg Lifts (61)** - 10 repetitions each side
- **Wall Assisted Pistol Squat (82)** - 5 repetitions each side
- **Wall Supported Hamstring Curl (62)** - 10 repetitions
- **Wall Assisted Calf Raises (24)** - 15 repetitions
- **Cool-Down:**
    - **Wall Supported Child's Pose (29)** - 3 minutes

Week 4: Upper Body and Balance

Weekly Goal: Strengthen upper body muscles and improve balance through varied exercises.

Daily Routine (10 minutes):

Pause for 20-30 seconds before moving on to the next exercise

- **Warm-Up:**
  - **Wall Chest Opener (10)** - 3 minutes
- **Wall Push-Up (17)** - 10 repetitions
- **Wall Supported Side Plank (25)** - Hold for 20 seconds each side
- **Wall Triangle Pose (32)** - Hold for 20 seconds each side
- **Wall Warrior Pose (33)** - Hold for 20 seconds each side
- **Wall Supported Balance Challenge (39)** - 10 repetitions
- **Wall Pike (48)** - Hold for 20 seconds
- **Cool-Down:**
  - **Wall Supported Relaxation (27)** - 3 minutes

Scan for Video!

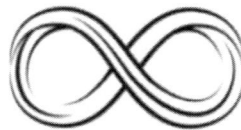

5.3 – For Advanced

Scan for Video!

Week 1: Advanced Core Activation

Weekly Goal: Challenge the core with advanced exercises for enhanced stability and strength.

Daily Routine (10 minutes):

Pause for 20-30 seconds before moving on to the next exercise

- **Warm-Up:**
  - **Wall Supported Hundred (2)** - 3 minutes
- **Wall Supported Plank with Leg Raise (37)** - 10 repetitions each side
- **Wall Supported Pike Press (58)** - 5 repetitions
- **Wall Supported Boat Pose Twist (59)** - 10 repetitions
- **Wall Climbing Stretch (81)** - Hold for 20 seconds
- **Wall Supported Leg Lifts (61)** - 10 repetitions each side
- **Wall Oblique Twists (52)** - 10 repetitions each side
- **Cool-Down:**
  - **Wall Supported Child's Pose (29)** - 3 minutes

Week 2: Enhancing Flexibility and Balance

Weekly Goal: Focus on improving flexibility and balance with challenging poses and stretches.

Daily Routine (10 minutes):

Pause for 20-30 seconds before moving on to the next exercise

Scan for Video!

- **Warm-Up:**
  - **Wall Downward Dog (14)** - 3 minutes
- **Wall Supported Split Progression (90)** - Hold for 20 seconds each side
- **Wall Assisted Forward Fold (80)** - Hold for 20 seconds
- **Wall Supported Side Kick Series (79)** - 5 repetitions each side
- **Wall Supported Warrior II (44)** - Hold for 20 seconds each side
- **Wall Triangle Pose (32)** - Hold for 20 seconds each side
- **Wall Supported Hip External Rotation Stretch (67)** - Hold for 20 seconds each side
- **Cool-Down:**
  - **Wall Supported Relaxation (27)** - 3 minutes

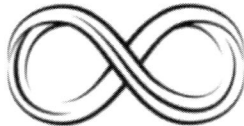

Week 3: Total Body Strength

Weekly Goal: Build total body strength with a focus on upper body, lower body, and dynamic movements.

Daily Routine (10 minutes):

Pause for 20-30 seconds before moving on to the next exercise

Scan for Video!

- **Warm-Up:**
  - **Wall Push-Up (17)** - 3 minutes
- **Wall Inverted Shoulder Press (88)** - 5 repetitions
- **Wall Supported Hamstring Curl (62)** - 10 repetitions
- **Wall Assisted Pistol Squat (82)** - 5 repetitions each side
- **Wall Burpees (55)** - 5 repetitions
- **Wall Diamond Push-Up (87)** - 5 repetitions
- **Wall Pike Slides (50)** - 10 repetitions
- **Cool-Down:**
  - **Wall Supported Fish Pose (28)** - 3 minutes

Week 4: Mastery of Movement and Mindfulness

Weekly Goal: Achieve mastery in movement through advanced exercises and enhance mindfulness.

Scan for Video!

Daily Routine (10 minutes):

Pause for 20-30 seconds before moving on to the next exercise

- **Warm-Up:**
    - **Wall Supported Bridge Lift (56)** - 3 minutes
- **Wall Supported Headstand (57)** - Hold for 20 seconds
- **Wall Supported Mermaid Pose (49)** - Hold for 20 seconds each side
- **Wall Supported Leg Raise with Rotation (70)** - 10 repetitions each side
- **Wall Supported Pike Stretch (60)** - Hold for 20 seconds
- **Wall Assisted Corkscrew (89)** - 10 repetitions each side
- **Wall Supported Side Stretch (83)** - Hold for 20 seconds each side
- **Cool-Down:**
    - **Wall Supported Relaxation (27)** - 3 minutes

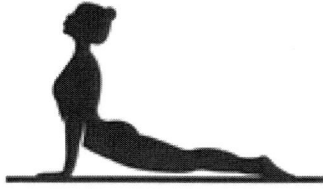

Chapter 6:

28-Day Challenge to Lose Weight

"You are only as young as your spine is flexible."

Joseph Pilates

Ready to kickstart your weight loss journey in a month?

This challenge is aimed at helping you shed pounds, improve heart health, and increase metabolism. Over 28 days, you'll follow a daily routine of exercises adaptable to your fitness level.

6.1 – For Beginners

Scan for Video!

Week 1: Introduction to Cardio and Strength Weekly Goal: Kickstart weight loss with a blend of basic cardio and strength exercises to boost metabolism.

Daily Routine (20 minutes):

Pause for 20-30 seconds before moving on to the next exercise

- **Warm-Up:**
  - **Wall Arm Slides (9)** - 2 minutes
- **Wall Supported Hundred (2)** - 2 minutes
- **Wall Sit with Leg Raise (18)** - 2 minutes (1 minute each leg)
- **Wall Push-Up (17)** - 2 minutes
- **Wall Plank (15)** - 2 minutes
- **Cool-Down:**
  - **Wall Supported Child's Pose (29)** - 3 minutes
  - **Wall Supported Relaxation (27)** - 2 minutes

Week 2: Building Endurance Weekly Goal: Increase endurance with longer holds and more repetitions to enhance calorie burn.

Scan for Video!

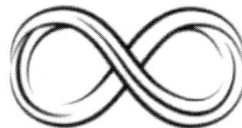

Daily Routine (20 minutes):

Pause for 20-30 seconds before moving on to the next exercise

- **Warm-Up:**
    - **Wall Shoulder Rolls (11)** - 2 minutes
- **Deep Wall Sit (8)** - 3 minutes
- **Wall Supported Bridge (7)** - 2 minutes
- **Wall Standing Leg Circles (5)** - 2 minutes (1 minute each leg)
- **Cool-Down:**
    - **Wall Supported Spinal Twist (30)** - 3 minutes
    - **Wall Supported Relaxation (27)** - 3 minutes

Week 3: Enhancing Flexibility and Mobility Weekly Goal: Improve flexibility and mobility to support efficient movement and prevent injuries.

Scan for Video!

Daily Routine (20 minutes):

Pause for 20-30 seconds before moving on to the next exercise

- **Warm-Up:**
    - **Wall Neck Extensions (12)** - 2 minutes
- **Wall Butterfly Stretch (20)** - 2 minutes
- **Wall Supported Ankle Stretches (22)** - 2 minutes
- **Wall Hamstring Stretch (16)** - 2 minutes (1 minute each side)
- **Cool-Down:**
    - **Wall Supported Fish Pose (28)** - 3 minutes
    - **Wall Supported Child's Pose (29)** - 3 minutes

Week 4: Core Focus and Stability Weekly Goal: Strengthen the core and improve stability, essential for overall fitness and effective weight loss.

Scan for Video!

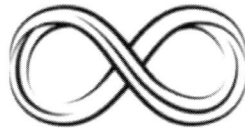

Daily Routine (20 minutes):

Pause for 20-30 seconds before moving on to the next exercise

- **Warm-Up:**
    - **Wall Pelvic Tilt (13)** - 2 minutes
- **Wall Reverse Plank (6)** - 2 minutes
- **Wall Supported Side Plank (25)** - 2 minutes (1 minute each side)
- **Wall Supported Bridge (7)** - 2 minutes
- **Cool-Down:**
    - **Wall Supported Relaxation (27)** - 3 minutes
    - **Wall Supported Child's Pose (29)** - 3 minutes

∞

6.2 – For Intermediate

Week 1: Intensifying Cardio and Strength Weekly Goal: Ramp up the intensity with a combination of intermediate cardio and strength exercises.

Scan for Video!

Daily Routine (20 minutes):

Pause for 20-30 seconds before moving on to the next exercise

- **Warm-Up:**
    - **Wall Arm Slides (9)** - 2 minutes
- **Wall Mountain Climbers (40)** - 2 minutes
- **Wall Supported Plank with Leg Raise (37)** - 2 minutes
- **Wall Oblique Twists (52)** - 2 minutes
- **Wall Supported Core Workout (38)** - 2 minutes
- **Cool-Down:**
    - **Wall Supported Spinal Twist (30)** - 3 minutes
    - **Wall Supported Relaxation (27)** - 2 minutes

Week 2: Advanced Endurance and Flexibility Weekly Goal: Focus on longer duration and more challenging exercises to further enhance endurance and flexibility.

Scan for Video!

Daily Routine (20 minutes):

Pause for 20-30 seconds before moving on to the next exercise

- **Warm-Up:**
  - **Wall Neck Extensions (12)** - 2 minutes
- **Wall Pigeon Pose (34)** - 2 minutes
- **Wall Supported Warrior II (44)** - 2 minutes
- **Wall Supported Hamstring Stretch (16)** - 2 minutes (1 minute each side)
- **Cool-Down:**
  - **Wall Supported Child's Pose (29)** - 3 minutes
  - **Wall Supported Fish Pose (28)** - 3 minutes

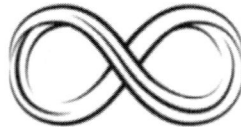

∞

Week 3: Building Dynamic Strength Weekly Goal: Incorporate dynamic movements to build strength and burn calories efficiently.

Scan for Video!

Daily Routine (20 minutes):

Pause for 20-30 seconds before moving on to the next exercise

Warm-Up:
  - **Wall Shoulder Rolls (11)** - 2 minutes

Wall Flutter Kicks (42) - 2 minutes

Wall Scissor Kicks (41) - 2 minutes

Wall Supported Squat Slide (45) - 2 minutes

Cool-Down:
  - **Wall Supported Spinal Twist (30)** - 3 minutes
  - **Wall Supported Relaxation (27)** - 3 minutes

Week 4: Balance and Core Stability Weekly Goal: Enhance balance and core stability for improved performance and efficient weight loss.

Scan for Video!

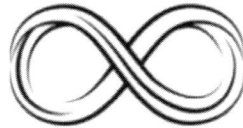

Daily Routine (20 minutes):

Pause for 20-30 seconds before moving on to the next exercise

- **Warm-Up:**

    - **Wall Pelvic Tilt (13)** - 2 minutes

- **Wall Triangle Pose (32)** - 2 minutes

- **Wall Supported Balance Challenge (39)** - 2 minutes

- **Wall Supported Leg Lifts (61)** - 2 minutes

- **Cool-Down:**

    - **Wall Supported Fish Pose (28)** - 3 minutes

    - **Wall Supported Child's Pose (29)** - 3 minutes

6.3 – For Advanced

Week 1: High-Intensity Cardio and Strength Weekly Goal: Maximize calorie burn with high-intensity cardio and strength exercises for advanced fitness levels.

Scan for Video!

Daily Routine (20 minutes):

Pause for 20-30 seconds before moving on to the next exercise

- **Warm-Up:**

    - **Wall Arm Slides (9)** - 2 minutes

- **Wall Burpees (55)** - 2 minutes

- **Wall Tuck Jumps (54)** - 2 minutes

Wall Supported Headstand (57) - 2 minutes

Cool-Down:

- **Wall Supported Pike Stretch (60)** - 3 minutes

- **Wall Supported Relaxation (27)** - 3 minutes

Week 2: Peak Endurance and Flexibility Weekly Goal: Push endurance and flexibility to the limit with challenging exercises.

Scan for Video!

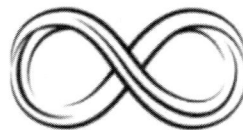

Daily Routine (20 minutes):

Pause for 20-30 seconds before moving on to the next exercise

- **Warm-Up:**

  - **Wall Neck Extensions (12)** - 2 minutes

- **Wall Assisted Pistol Squat (82)** - 2 minutes

- **Wall Supported Hip Abductor Stretch (64)** - 2 minutes

- **Wall Supported Boat Pose Twist (59)** - 2 minutes

- **Cool-Down:**

  - **Wall Supported Child's Pose (29)** - 3 minutes

  - **Wall Supported Fish Pose (28)** - 3 minutes

∞

Week 3: Advanced Dynamic Strength Weekly Goal: Focus on advanced dynamic strength exercises for maximum efficiency in weight loss.

Scan for Video!

Daily Routine (20 minutes):

Pause for 20-30 seconds before moving on to the next exercise

- **Warm-Up:**

  - **Wall Shoulder Rolls (11)** - 2 minutes

- **Wall Inverted Shoulder Press (88)** - 2 minutes

- **Wall Diamond Push-Up (87)** - 2 minutes

- **Wall Supported Hamstring Curl (62)** - 2 minutes

- **Cool-Down:**

  - **Wall Supported Spinal Twist (30)** - 3 minutes

  - **Wall Supported Relaxation (27)** - 3 minutes

Week 4: Ultimate Balance and Core Stability Weekly Goal: Achieve ultimate balance and core stability with advanced exercises.

Scan for Video!

Daily Routine (20 minutes):

Pause for 20-30 seconds before moving on to the next exercise

- **Warm-Up:**

    - **Wall Pelvic Tilt (13)** - 2 minutes

Wall Climbing Stretch (81) - 2 minutes

Wall Supported Leg Raise with Rotation (70) - 2 minutes

Wall Supported Hip Hinge with Leg Lift (91) - 2 minutes

Cool-Down:

- **Wall Supported Fish Pose (28)** - 3 minutes

- **Wall Supported Child's Pose (29)** - 3 minutes

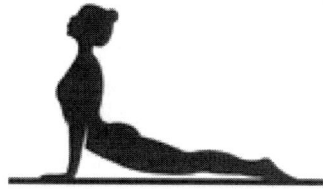

CHAPTER 7:

11 HEALTHY TIPS TO BOOST YOUR FITNESS RESULTS

"True flexibility can be achieved only when all muscles are uniformly developed."

Joseph Pilates

Embarking on a Wall Pilates journey as a senior is a commendable step towards enhancing your overall well-being. But did you know that coupling your exercise regimen with certain lifestyle habits can significantly amplify your fitness results? Here's a deep dive into some healthy lifestyle tips that complement your Wall Pilates practice, ensuring you get the most out of your efforts.

1. **Why Is Hydration So Crucial for Fitness?**

   Hydration plays a pivotal role in maintaining optimal body function, especially during exercise. Drinking enough water helps to:

   - Improve Joint Lubrication: Adequate hydration ensures your joints are well-lubricated, reducing the risk of injury during your Wall Pilates sessions.

   - Enhance Muscle Performance: Muscles that are well-hydrated perform better, allowing for a more effective workout.

   - Boost Recovery: Water aids in flushing out toxins, speeding up the recovery process after exercise.

2. **How Does a Balanced Diet Impact Your Pilates Practice?**

   A balanced diet fuels your body with the essential nutrients it needs to perform at its best. Integrating a variety of fruits, vegetables, lean proteins, and whole grains into your diet can:

   - Provide Sustained Energy: Proper nutrition ensures you have the energy to complete your Pilates routine and engage in daily activities.

   - Support Muscle Repair and Growth: Protein-rich foods aid in muscle recovery and growth, essential for building strength through Wall Pilates.

- Enhance Flexibility and Mobility: Foods rich in omega-3 fatty acids, such as fish and nuts, can improve flexibility and reduce inflammation.

3. **Why Should You Prioritize Sleep and How Does It Affect Your Fitness?**

Quality sleep is paramount for anyone looking to improve their fitness. A good night's sleep can:

- Enhance Recovery: Sleep is when your body repairs itself. Getting enough rest allows your muscles to heal and strengthen.

- Boost Energy Levels: Well-rested individuals have more energy to put into their workouts, resulting in more productive sessions.

- Improve Focus: Adequate sleep improves cognitive function, helping you stay focused during your Wall Pilates exercises.

4. **What Role Does Stress Management Play in Achieving Fitness Goals?**

Stress can have a detrimental effect on your fitness journey by:

- Impairing Recovery: High stress levels can impede your body's ability to recover from exercise.

- Reducing Motivation: Stress can lower your motivation to exercise and lead a healthy lifestyle.

- Affecting Sleep: Stress often leads to sleep disturbances, further impacting your fitness progress. Incorporating stress-reducing activities such as meditation, deep breathing exercises, or even gentle walks can help manage stress levels, complementing your Wall Pilates practice.

5. **How Important Is Consistency in Your Exercise Routine?**

Consistency is key to seeing progress in any fitness regimen. Regularly practicing Wall Pilates:

Builds Muscle Memory: Consistent practice helps your body adapt to the exercises, improving form and efficiency over time.

Enhances Long-term Results: Steady, gradual improvements lead to more significant, long-lasting fitness outcomes.

Boosts Mental Well-being: Regular exercise contributes to better mental health, reducing symptoms of depression and anxiety.

6. **Why Choose a Holistic Approach with Wall Pilates?**

Wall Pilates transcends traditional physical exercise by embracing a holistic approach that nurtures mind, body, and spirit. This practice:

- **Fosters Physical and Mental Harmony**: Integrating Wall Pilates into your daily routine helps in aligning your physical movements with your breath, creating a harmonious balance between body and mind.

- **Reduces Stress and Enhances Focus:** Regular practice helps in significantly lowering stress levels while sharpening mental focus, making it easier to navigate daily challenges.

- **Strengthens Emotional Resilience**: By promoting mindfulness and self-awareness, Wall Pilates builds a strong foundation for emotional resilience, aiding in better management of life's ups and downs.

7. **How Can I Tailor Wall Pilates to Fit My Life?**

    The beauty of Wall Pilates lies in its adaptability to fit any lifestyle or schedule. Tailoring your practice can be achieved by:

    - **Creating Customizable Routines**: Whether you have 15 minutes or an hour, you can design your Wall Pilates session to fit into your day, ensuring that you consistently benefit from your practice.

    - **Adapting to Energy Levels**: Select routines that match your energy levels at different times of the day, whether it's a vigorous morning session to boost your day or a gentle evening routine for relaxation.

    - **Emphasizing Consistency Over Duration**: Even short, regular sessions can lead to significant improvements in flexibility, strength, and mental well-being, underscoring the importance of making Wall Pilates a consistent part of your life.

8. **Is it Possible to Feel a Sense of Community Through Wall Pilates?**

    Absolutely. Wall Pilates offers a unique opportunity to connect with a supportive community, whether online or in-person. This connection:

    - **Encourages Shared Experiences**: Participating in group classes or online forums allows for the sharing of experiences, tips, and encouragement, fostering a sense of belonging and motivation.

    - **Provides Motivation and Support**: The camaraderie found in Wall Pilates communities can be a powerful motivator, helping you to stay committed to your practice and achieve your fitness goals.

    - **Enhances Learning and Growth**: Being part of a community gives you access to a wealth of collective knowledge, enabling you to learn new techniques and deepen your practice.

9. **Can Wall Pilates Help with Mindfulness and Relaxation?**

    Incorporating mindfulness into your Wall Pilates practice can profoundly enhance its benefits, including:

    - **Promoting Deep Relaxation**: Focusing on breath and movement helps in activating the body's relaxation response, reducing stress and promoting a state of calm.

    - **Improving Mind-Body Connection**: Mindfulness during Wall Pilates strengthens the connection between mind and body, enhancing awareness and control over your physical state.

    - **Boosting Mental Clarity**: The meditative aspects of mindful Wall Pilates practice can clear the mind, improve concentration, and foster a sense of inner peace.

10. How Do I Make Wall Pilates a Part of My Lifestyle?

Integrating Wall Pilates into your lifestyle requires a dedicated approach, including:

- **Designing a Dedicated Space**: Create a specific area in your home for your Wall Pilates practice, making it inviting and easily accessible to encourage regular use.

- **Setting Achievable Goals**: Define clear, achievable goals related to your Wall Pilates practice, such as increasing flexibility or strength, to keep motivated and on track.

- **Tracking Progress**: Maintain a journal or log of your Wall Pilates sessions and any improvements you notice in your physical and mental well-being to motivate continued practice.

11. What About Nurturing Growth and Adaptability in My Practice?

As you progress in your Wall Pilates journey, it's essential to nurture growth and remain adaptable by:

- **Exploring Advanced Techniques**: As your strength and flexibility improve, incorporate more challenging poses and sequences to continuously advance your practice.

- **Listening to Your Body**: Adapt your practice based on your body's changing needs and limitations, ensuring a safe and effective workout.

- **Staying Open to Learning**: Embrace new learning opportunities, whether through workshops or online resources, to enhance your understanding and execution of Wall Pilates.

CONCLUSION AND THANKS

When our joint story comes to an end, let's pause to reflect on the adventure we have traveled together. This book is more than just an anthology of methods and exercises; it's a portal to an infinite universe of possibilities that illuminates a route full of wellness, balance, and peace. Our journey doesn't finish here. Rather, it's the beginning of an amazing journey to fully embrace life, every moment of conscious presence, every breath, and every stretch.

To you, the reader,

who has ventured to welcome the practice of Wall Pilates

and its vast advantages into your life,

I offer my profoundest thanks.

It is with sincere hope that this volume acts as your beacon of joy,

a fountain of peace, and a trigger for active physical participation,

bringing a harmonious balance into your existence.

May the techniques unveiled within inspire you

to tap into your inherent strength and agility,

to find the stable ground within yourself,

and to release the dynamic energy that fuels your every deed.

Continue to discover, to extend, and to glow.

Your finest moments are not in the past;

they are blossoming at this very moment,

with every breath you draw and every posture you assume

in your Wall Pilates practice.

Yours sincerely,
Grace Noren

MONTHLY HEALTHY PLANNER

MONTH OF :

S
Date	Wall Pilates			Date	Wall Pilates			Date	Wall Pilates			Date	Wall Pilates			Date	Wall Pilates		
	Yes	No			Yes	No			Yes	No			Yes	No			Yes	No	
Hrs.Slept				Hrs.Slept				Hrs.Slept				Hrs.Slept				Hrs.Slept			
Diet				Diet				Diet				Diet				Diet			
Water Glas.				Water Glas.				Water Glas.				Water Glas.				Water Glas.			

M
Date	Wall Pilates			Date	Wall Pilates			Date	Wall Pilates			Date	Wall Pilates			Date	Wall Pilates		
	Yes	No			Yes	No			Yes	No			Yes	No			Yes	No	
Hrs.Slept				Hrs.Slept				Hrs.Slept				Hrs.Slept				Hrs.Slept			
Diet				Diet				Diet				Diet				Diet			
Water Glas.				Water Glas.				Water Glas.				Water Glas.				Water Glas.			

T
Date	Wall Pilates			Date	Wall Pilates			Date	Wall Pilates			Date	Wall Pilates			Date	Wall Pilates		
	Yes	No			Yes	No			Yes	No			Yes	No			Yes	No	
Hrs.Slept				Hrs.Slept				Hrs.Slept				Hrs.Slept				Hrs.Slept			
Diet				Diet				Diet				Diet				Diet			
Water Glas.				Water Glas.				Water Glas.				Water Glas.				Water Glas.			

W
Date	Wall Pilates			Date	Wall Pilates			Date	Wall Pilates			Date	Wall Pilates			Date	Wall Pilates		
	Yes	No			Yes	No			Yes	No			Yes	No			Yes	No	
Hrs.Slept				Hrs.Slept				Hrs.Slept				Hrs.Slept				Hrs.Slept			
Diet				Diet				Diet				Diet				Diet			
Water Glas.				Water Glas.				Water Glas.				Water Glas.				Water Glas.			

T
Date	Wall Pilates			Date	Wall Pilates			Date	Wall Pilates			Date	Wall Pilates			Date	Wall Pilates		
	Yes	No			Yes	No			Yes	No			Yes	No			Yes	No	
Hrs.Slept				Hrs.Slept				Hrs.Slept				Hrs.Slept				Hrs.Slept			
Diet				Diet				Diet				Diet				Diet			
Water Glas.				Water Glas.				Water Glas.				Water Glas.				Water Glas.			

F
Date	Wall Pilates			Date	Wall Pilates			Date	Wall Pilates			Date	Wall Pilates			Date	Wall Pilates		
	Yes	No			Yes	No			Yes	No			Yes	No			Yes	No	
Hrs.Slept				Hrs.Slept				Hrs.Slept				Hrs.Slept				Hrs.Slept			
Diet				Diet				Diet				Diet				Diet			
Water Glas.				Water Glas.				Water Glas.				Water Glas.				Water Glas.			

S
Date	Wall Pilates			Date	Wall Pilates			Date	Wall Pilates			Date	Wall Pilates			Date	Wall Pilates		
	Yes	No			Yes	No			Yes	No			Yes	No			Yes	No	
Hrs.Slept				Hrs.Slept				Hrs.Slept				Hrs.Slept				Hrs.Slept			
Diet				Diet				Diet				Diet				Diet			
Water Glas.				Water Glas.				Water Glas.				Water Glas.				Water Glas.			

SCAN HERE!

SCAN THIS QR-CODE
TO PRINT THE PLANNER

ABOUT THE AUTHOR

Grace Noren stands as a testament to the transformative and healing power of introspection, resilience, and the ancient practices of Yoga and Pilates. Her journey from an elementary school teacher to a revered personal instructor for seniors is not just a career shift but a profound voyage into the depths of emotional and physical healing, driven by a deeply personal experience that reshaped her understanding of wellness and compassion.

Grace's life took a pivotal turn when her mother, at 64, faced a debilitating injury that confined her to bed for an agonizing three months. This period of helplessness and despair brought Grace face to face with the limitations of conventional healing methods and led her to the gentle embrace of Chair yoga, Wall Pilates and Somatics. These practices became a beacon of hope, not just for her mother, who began to show signs of recovery and newfound strength, but for Grace herself, who found in it a calling that resonated with her soul.

This experience awakened in Grace a profound sense of purpose and a deep-seated passion for the healing arts. She embarked on an intensive study of Yoga, Pilates, and Somatics embracing these practices not only as physical exercises but as pathways to inner peace and emotional resilience. Her transition from a teacher of young children to a personal instructor for seniors reflects a journey marked by empathy, patience, and an unwavering commitment to nurturing the well-being of others.

Today, Grace's sessions are more than just fitness classes; they are intimate gatherings where emotions are acknowledged, vulnerabilities are embraced, and every movement is an act of self-care and love.

Made in United States
North Haven, CT
01 July 2024

54270298R00065